CONTENTS

Mistress Pussycat

Adventures With Submissive Men
In The World Of Femdom

an investigate memoir
by Joyce Snyder

A Headpress Book

for my brokerage account

AUTHOR'S NOTE

THIS IS A TRUE STORY. AMONG THE MANY MEN described within these pages, there are no composite characters—their actions and proclivities are individual. However, specific characteristics and possible identifiers have been altered to assure a person's privacy. Physical descriptions of males are purposely kept vague; but all body types mentioned are accurate. Domiciles and professions of these men have been changed, except for those I met at DomSubFriends Speed Dating. I've kept a few facts intact: I have not misrepresented any man's relative wealth and social standing. When profiling someone, if his religion is mentioned, then this is also true. Also faithfully represented is a man's current marital status—if it is stated that he's single and not married, he is exactly that.

For people detailed in this book, I have changed most—not all—real names as well as scene names (used in the lifestyle). When I've done so, an asterisk has been placed by a name the first time it is used.

Thank you, Robert Rosen, for suggesting I contact your savvy publisher, David Kerekes at Headpress. More thanks to attorneys Stephen Perretta for his assistance and Corrine Irish for her legal review. Kudos to Sonja Wagner for shooting my perfect book cover. I'd like to acknowledge The Eulenspiegel Society for their cooperation and continued good work. And much gratitude to the submissive men I've met for allowing me into their world.

ONE

Women Enslaving Men? Why Not!

SIXTY WAS THE ADOLESCENCE OF MY OLD AGE, time to try new things. I was already well traveled, but in my sixtieth year I would visit some long-anticipated places—Poland, Vienna, Chile. With my three cats in tow, I'd recently moved from a rental into a co-op (both one-bedrooms in Manhattan's Chelsea). I would perfect my bridge game and add some rare beauties to my vintage perfume collection. I still dated, but sporadically; age plus past experience had made me as picky as my prospects. My dismal job of 30 years' standing involved working for big porn publishers. One positive thing resulted from this disreputable career path—I finally discovered my true sexuality, and in the seventh decade of my life.

Leg Action was among a handful of magazines I was newly assigned to edit. For over two decades, the title had featured pictorials, letters and stories involving tall, leggy, cruel dominant women. I had long known about "dommes," those severe, commanding women in stiletto heels, leather and corselets who ruled over men and were often generously compensated for doing so. But I'd given little thought to submissive men, having no idea what made them submit to dominant women, or believe women were the superior gender. And why they enjoyed having women tease, humiliate, control, or inflict pain upon them—often even paying these dommes for it! But since it was suddenly my duty to entertain, inform and sexually satisfy a readership of submissive men, I decided to better educate myself about dominant females and the men who craved them. No one at work suggested I actively participate in any research. My only instructions were to "go after the competition." (At the time, there was another, more established magazine, also sold on the newsstand, featuring leggy dominant women.)

I realized that "femdom," as female dominance is called in popular culture, was an important part of the entire BDSM scene. (BDSM is the acronym derived from *bondage* and *discipline* plus *sadism* and *masochism.*) In femdom, a woman assumes the dominant role in bondage, discipline and sadistic play, which is why she is termed a dominatrix, domina or domme. Similarly, for female submissives, the man who dominates them is a *dom.*

In New York City circa 2010, meetings, workshops, lectures and parties were sponsored by several such organizations, including DomSubFriends, The Eulenspiegel Society, and ClubFEM. Most get togethers were mere blocks away from where I lived in Chelsea, a neighborhood those in the scene regarded as Manhattan's kink central. The New York City based DomSubFriends was soon to have a speed dating event at Manhattan's premier BDSM joint, Paddles. Although this subterranean club with a dungeon motif was located close to my home, I'd never been there.

Speed dating, I laughed to myself, as I walked over to Paddles. I had never attended such an event, though I was too old to ever have participated. Invented in 1998 by a rabbi, specifically to get Jewish girls in front of many Jewish boys, these forced meetings were designed to result in a match. But as an instrument of romance (and preventer of intermarriage) speed dating at Jewish singles events was sorely lacking. The women were seated while the men moved from one female to the next. Both parties interrogated each other about jobs held, colleges attended, cars driven, homes owned and, of course, their religious practice and level of observance. After each sized the other up, a bell would ring to signal the end of conversation. *Next!* Since its beginnings, the speed dating ritual has been widely practiced in many cultures all over the world. But how could such basic summaries translate to a milieu as complex as BDSM? And was it even possible that a dominant woman could, in mere minutes, measure the murky motivations of a submissive man?

The BDSM community is well-organized, as was the DomSub-Friends speed dating event. Before it began, on first entering the underground club Paddles, I was approached by several dominant fellows who were immediately open and friendly. They'd begin a very general conversation, then shortly and abruptly ask "are you a bottom?" When I disclosed I was a domme, not a submissive, they were not interested in continuing our chat. The guys I met at Paddles were there for a reason—to find compatible play partners.

Paddles had strict no penetration and no ejaculation rules, plus "dungeon monitors" who made sure all activities were safe and within their guidelines. There one could be bound and strung up in a spiderweb of ropes, have their bottom beaten raw with a cane or become ground zero for a series of electric jolts—yet no liquid deposit was permitted. These rules existed so Paddles could remain open as a meeting and play space for the New York City area's BDSM community. At the time of my visit, Paddles had been operating for over 30 years. I couldn't think of one Manhattan nightclub with that track record.

We speed daters were soon broken up into groups. "All dominant men and submissive women meet by the bar!" an organizer bellowed. I could now tell the difference between the leather-clad dominant men and the submissive guys, those who wore more conservative, casual street clothes. The submissive women, in high heels and short skirts, were all younger and thinner than we dominant women who, with the submissive men, were herded into a cave-like dungeon.

Of the roughly 30 attendees, about half were now in this room. I had no idea if there was a submissive woman for every dominant man in the bar area, but in the grotto there were precisely seven sub guys for seven dommes. This observation had the group moderator, the fortyish Master Dan*, recall the old movie musical *Seven Brides For Seven Brothers*.

I was, by far, the oldest (at age 60) and thinnest (112 pounds) woman present. We were then given blank name tags to fill in, so we could be identified and addressed. I noticed how doms (like Master Dan) were addressed as Sir or Master, while dommes put Lady or Mistress before their names.

"All dommes, please be seated and submissive men, get on your knees!" shouted Master Dan, gesturing with a well-toned arm in the direction of some oddly shaped seats. I made a beeline for a padded bench which resembled gym equipment and sat there, happy I'd be receiving my submissives in comfort.

"You've got four minutes before we ring a bell and the subs, still on your knees, will then move on to the next domme. After you've spoken with everyone of the opposite sex, you'll write down, in order of preference, who you'd like to play with tonight. Got it?" As he explained the brief speed dating rules, Master Dan distributed a piece of paper with a blank line after the word *your name* and spaces to write down others' names and take notes. "Rate only 1-5 (high best)" was printed on the handout. We were each ranking the other in order to be matched, as they did in regular speed dating. Unlike the vanilla speed dates, any mutual interest would not result in phone numbers exchanged or future dates but immediate dirty dungeon doings. I had no idea what this entailed, but taking in the bondage beds, leather spanking benches, metal cages, thick wooden paddles, piles of twisted ropes and chains—I knew this old bride wasn't ready to meet and beat any brother!

The first fellow was now before me on bended knees, staring up at me only briefly, specifically to focus on my name tag. "Hello, Mistress Joyce," a forty-something well-built fellow began softly, his head bowed in what was either shyness or mock respect. None of the guys ever looked at a domme directly—eye contact was a definite breach of submissive etiquette.

"Hello Gary*," I replied briskly. "Tell me what turns you on."

"I like it when the woman is on top." He spoke with no hesitation and complete confidence. "I'm heavy into body worship as well as smothering."

I didn't exactly know what was involved in body worship. And the smothering mention brought to mind this bizarre image of a man I had briefly dated decades ago, the author Jerzy Kosinski, who had killed himself by placing a plastic bag over his head. "How do these activities make you feel?"

"It makes me feel whole to revere a woman." His voice was even and measured.

"So, what else do you like to do?" I asked in the peppy manner single vanilla speed daters affect.

"Mummification," he answered with a calm certainty.

"O.K. What do you do for work?"

"I'm a massage therapist."

Before I could fathom the temptations such an erotically charged job presented, our four minutes together were up. Gary, still kneeling, now crept a foot or two over, presenting himself before the domme seated beside me.

The next sub, Jerry*, was a clean-cut, well dressed dude in his mid-thirties who confessed his sexuality revolved around "step-stool humiliation." I had no idea how a man could be humiliated with a step-stool or why he'd even want to be. Jerry worked in finance and lived downtown. I quickly scribbled on my paper score pad other things Jerry claimed to enjoy: having his nipples pinched, being hit or slapped, a woman spitting in his open mouth, trampling, and ass smothering.

"What's your kind of play partner?"

"An open-minded domme who can easily and naturally assume her superiority. And one who dishes out lots of verbal humiliation."

"Why?"

"*Why*?" he repeated my question. "Because," he hesitated for just a second before blurting, "I need to feel lower than the woman I'm with." I could imagine this Wall Streeter later returning home to his multi-million dollar downtown loft. Before I could probe further, there was that bell again.

Donald*, a doctor in a busy urban hospital, next lumbered over on his knees. He explained how in his job he always had to be in control.

But during his off-hours and erotic life, Donald craved the feeling that came with being out of control—resulting in a sexual release. "I'm open to things," he acknowledged, without getting into specifics. "But what turns me on most of all is the power exchange."

The man who followed confessed he liked the feeling of "being toyed with." The guy after him could handle heavy duty sadistic play but "wasn't into strap-ons." A few claimed they needed to feel *forced* to participate in activities such as smothering and trampling. All sought a strong, authoritative woman who could dish out the pain and humiliation they craved. A confident, naturally sadistic domme would erase the burden of asking for such treatment.

"I have to feed my cats now," I whispered to Master Dan, after seeing my seventh and final sub, then dashed out of Paddles before the matching results were tallied. I cared little whether any ranked me high or low—they were all two decades too young. But what if I had been forty years old instead of sixty? Sizing them up, these fellows were equal to what I'd randomly find on the Match website or in a singles bar. None were outwardly kinky in looks or demeanor. Instead, they appeared as standard-issue guys who thought they deserved to find what they wanted. They might be looking for a woman to spit in their open mouth instead of a perfect ten or a high wage earner, but at least they seemed honest and self-aware.

I won't engage in that kind of erotic play until I have it down cold, I convinced myself, as I walked home in the balmy spring night. The moves, the attitude, the philosophy must be certain and innate. These men don't deserve a tremulous and unsure sex partner. They want a forceful bitch goddess who lives and breathes female superiority—and I'm just not there! But surely a man who thinks himself a slave to women, a man who views women as the superior sex, had to be better than Glen*, the last guy I'd dated.

Glen, in his early seventies and father of grown children, had been divorced for at least a decade. A former financial type, he now consulted just enough to speak knowledgeably about the stock market, ask his decades younger date where she was invested, then write off the meal as a tax deduction. A female friend had fixed me up with him. "Look, it's just a dinner and he's totally harmless," she'd vouched. Dinner sounded good to me and harmless even better. We were to meet at an Upper East Side spot my girlfriend deemed "very social," noting its patrons skewed to an older demographic.

I greeted Glen, who was well-turned-out in a navy blue double-breasted blazer and charcoal slacks. His hair was a natural gray, without any gruesome dye job, and he had no obvious missing teeth. For a guy in his early seventies, he made an excellent impression. So far, so good, I thought as the waiter took our drink orders. But when Glen began to chit the chat, things quickly went downhill. Starting with current events, he zeroed in on the Tiger Woods cheating scandal, the predominant media morality play at the time. Leaning towards me, he offered this comment on the *affaire de jour*: "Tiger Woods has a big dick, I hear his girlfriend says, and he likes anal sex!"

I offered a feeble "my, my" in response before he went on to discuss politics. I've thankfully blanked from memory his exact comment, which had something to do with the President along those same lines. "You know, Glen, I hear enough about politics and current events. I'd like to know more about *you*."

"Well, I'm semi-retired, divorced for several years now, my PSA level is 2.8 and anything under 4 is desirable." In Manhattan perhaps, an older man's test results for prostate cancer had bragging rights along with his career, address and children's schools. "I live right here on the Upper East," he continued. "What about you?"

"I live in Chelsea."

"Do you live with anyone or are you alone?"

"I live with my three cats."

Glen chuckled. "Well, that's got to be a handful."

Maybe he wasn't so bad after all, I told myself, as I sipped a glass of Cabernet. "They're pretty easy, except I'm worried about one cat who's had a stroke."

"Don't say you're worried, say 'I have concern.' I have *concern* for my cat who has had a stroke."

"I'm not just concerned, I'm really worried," I confided.

"But that's negative and you can't be negative. Like your job?"

"*Uh-huh.*"

"What did you say you did? Graphic artist?"

I nodded. There was no way I was telling anyone I didn't know well how I'd worked as a pornographer these past three decades. Their highly colored reactions, rife with wild assumptions and negative judgments, were typically more than I could handle.

"Do you like to cook?" he asked.

"I recently moved into a new place. I like it, except there's not enough cabinet or counter space in the kitchen. I was planning to re-do my kitchen when I learned the co-op was soon replacing the heating pipes. So for now, I have several boxes stacked in my big eat-in kitchen because all renovations are temporarily on hold. That's the problem."

"Don't say *problem*, say *opportunity*," he reprimanded me. "I have an *opportunity* with my kitchen."

After more of the same psychobabble with some big dick talk sprinkled in, he suggested having a nightcap at his apartment nearby. To figure out a man, one need only take a peek at his premises and I was curious enough to follow him up the elevator.

"My next door neighbor is gay and has this really big dog. Sometimes he has another guy over and they have threesomes with the dog," Glen smirked, while turning his front door key. I knew what was coming. "And the dog has this really big dick!" he offered happily, his hands about a foot apart, as if measuring.

Now it was time for me to take *his* measure. I looked around the tiny one-bedroom apartment. A double bed dominated the living room; another such bed nearly filled the crowded bedroom. It appeared as if Glen did not live alone. When I saw one of those inspirational be-positive books on his coffee table, I surmised this guy had missed the lifeboat, was clutching at a lifesaver and going down fast. No drink for me, it was time to fake a tummy ache, bid a hasty *adieu* and beat it out of there! Taking a taxi home, I pondered whether a submissive man—one who allowed himself to be put in a collar, led on a leash and perform household duties in exchange for prolonged cunnilingus privileges—would be preferable to those older guys still available.

I had asked asked DomSubFriends' Master Dan where I could find submissive men in The Lifestyle who were older than his speed dating bunch. (Both BDSM and the partner-swapping swinging community are called "the lifestyle" in much the way that Hollywood, as well as the San Fernando Valley porn community, each refer to their frenetic commerce as "the business.") He'd directed me to ClubFEM, the only group specifically dedicated to female domination over male submissives. Or, as their slogan boldly declared under its abstract bustier logo, "Women Enslaving Men." The New York City branch was one of 21 (in the United States) in addition to 7 foreign-based active ClubFEM chapters. With a presence in such unsuspected female supremacy outposts as St. Louis, Missouri and Columbus, Ohio, ClubFEM ruled this burgeoning movement. Founded in 1992 by a bunch of bad-ass Texas broads, chapters bloomed in an intriguingly random pattern. Cowboys would congregate at ClubFEM Wyoming, that stronghold of unbridled masculinity, so that dommes could perhaps hogtie them as they would cattle. Three chapters were in Texas, a state known for its strong, conservative men and four more cropped up Down Under for rugged Australians. Social movements spring from where there is a social need—judging from the chapter geography, it seemed as though female domination was desired in the most macho local cultures.

BDSM devotees can connect outside a dungeon, or play space, in places other than the myriad websites geared to their participation. One time-honored tradition is the "munch," where dominants can meet submissive partners at a casual dining venue. In order to attend a ClubFEM munch, I first had to submit a letter of introduction—they demanded to know what kind of person was attending their event and why. In the spring of 2010, I sent an e-mail to Headmistress Reina at ClubFEM's New York City Chapter.

I would like to apply for membership in ClubFEM. I am a mature woman who has worked in porn for 30 years and never married. I hardly required a husband. But now I find myself interested in having a sub. I've a genuine inclination towards dominating men. In my professional life (as producer of several x-rated films) I've hardly been the shrinking violet. In my personal life (I've dated for decades) I was always encouraged by men not to assert myself or be demanding in any way. I railed against this, even as the slur "JAP" was flung at me. I live in Chelsea and am free to immerse myself in the ClubFEM lifestyle.

In Sisterhood,
Joyce Snyder

Her response detailed where their next munch would be held and reminded me women must first attend three gatherings to be membership-worthy. While perusing their website's event schedule, I noticed they held themed parties about every six weeks. Past events had included Caning, Objectification, Forced Feminization and Sensual Mummification. On the schedule for 2010 were Foot Worship, Pony Party, Strap-Ons and Medical Play.

Could wanting to please a female actually be a fetish? If so, there seemed to be countless men who existed solely to satisfy their woman. Her wishes were always paramount in their minds and the words "yes, dear" usually on their lips. But these men weren't kinksters, they were called *husbands*—and I didn't have one.

The munch was held at a coffee shop's back room filled with uncomfortable, hard chairs—something I avoided as much as marriage. (Soft seats were so important to me, I'd visited the place a few days before the event, just to check out their seating arrangements.) I entered the ClubFEM munch wearing a black *haori* (a knee-length version of a Japanese kimono) and carrying a shopping bag which contained a big pillow.

Over two dozen people at three long tables were already present. On my left sat an attractive fellow of approximately my age who introduced himself as Len*. He immediately inquired about the activities I enjoyed. This launched us into travel talk, specifically Eastern Europe, and we compared notes. I had previously assumed the typical submissive man would be somewhat reticent, with a bland countenance and unassuming presence. But Len was none of that—instead he was interesting and well-spoken. Plus he was divorced, with a credible job and house in the nearby New Jersey suburbs. I was intrigued to find out more.

After it was established this was my first ClubFEM activity, Len revealed where his own interests lie—sensory deprivation. He was eager for a sophisticated lady who would put him into a straightjacket, he confided, then assured me no sex play was involved. Len thought I would fit the bill nicely. I squirmed on my overstuffed square pillow. "So what exactly does the woman you're with do?"

"I have a cellar. You must force me down the stairs, blindfold me, put me in my straightjacket and make me crawl into the ice box. Naturally, some whipping is in order. Then you just go back upstairs to read or watch television in my big, comfortable home and wait a few hours."

"Wait for what?"

"For the ice to melt. See, I have a key embedded in the ice, very near where I can reach to unbind myself." He looked at me with an incredulous expression. "You didn't think I would actually keep the icebox *on*, did you?"

"It never even occurred to me. See, I'm still trying to process our proposed rendezvous—cellar, freezer, straightjacket, whip, key. I've got to admit, Len, I'm basically used to dinner or a movie."

"Think about it. Oh, that's Reina," he muttered, as ClubFEM's headmistress stood to address the assembled 19 submissive men and 11 dominant women.

Reina, which means *queen*, was a queen-sized young woman who possessed a natural air of authority mixed with good cheer. No one dared to speak over Headmistress Reina as she detailed upcoming events. She was poised, talking easily without written notes and with a good deal of charm. Her chat was spiked with peals of infectious wicked giggles when mentioning the play, rituals and humiliation ClubFEM slaves were soon to endure. Reina oozed self-confidence and was totally in command.

It was time for everyone to introduce themselves, explain their interests and why they were there. A man in his thirties, who sat on my right and at the end of the table, was the first to stand. "I'm Axel* and I'm owned by Lady Velour*. I'm called Xena* when I dress up as a woman; but when I play as a puppy I'm Tuffy*. And I'm a total slut!" he proudly concluded before sitting down to an appreciative round of applause.

Next it would be my turn. "You never say your real name," Len murmured in my ear. "Give us your scene name."

"I wasn't given one," I whispered back.

"Then make one up *now*."

I thought about the image on my pillow (a cat's face) and of the three cats I had at home, then stood before 30 pairs of appraising eyes. "Hello, I'm Mistress Pussycat. I'm into being demanding, complaining a lot, plus controlling and dominating men. I'm here to learn and also to find others who are supportive of my behavior." Some polite clapping followed as I sat down. Len spoke next, elaborating on his love of sensory deprivation in all its facets, which he found incredibly erotic.

At the evening's end, I was anticipating ClubFEM's next event, which was not a munch but a Pony Party. As I stood to leave, a man in his early forties approached me. "Mistress Pussycat, do you know yet what to do?" he asked with a pronounced European accent.

"Not yet, I'm just learning." He abruptly spun around to chat with a petite brunette and addressed her as Mistress Trish. She spoke in a low, measured tone somewhere between bored and I-mean-serious-business.

Remarking on this exchange, Len noted: "The guy needs discipline. If he can't get it from a newbie lifestyle domme like you, he'll seek out a pro-domme like Mistress Trish."

"What's the difference?"

"Pro-dommes charge money for BDSM sessions, humiliation, kink or just to be in the same room with them. Lifestyle dommes do it for free because that's where they're at, sexually, and because they love it."

"A few guys who spoke said they were "collared." What does that mean: they wear a collar?"

"Yes, sometimes they wear a collar but that's not necessary. It's like being married. When a collared man belongs to a domme, it's a monogamous relationship with serious responsibilities. Many collared subs are also legally married to their dommes. We have collaring rites just as there are marriage ceremonies in the vanilla world."

"*Vanilla* world? What is that?"

"We in BDSM refer to anything decidedly outside our world as vanilla.

"Can you use it in a sentence?"

"Sure. You could say: 'He was in the lifestyle but had a vanilla girlfriend. What kind of vanilla activities do you enjoy? We mustn't do anything too obviously kinky in public, it will freak out the vanilla.'"

"O.K., I get it. Vanilla is everyone and everything else." We were now on the sidewalk, preparing to go our separate ways.

"I'd like to see you again, Mistress Pussycat. You could put me in the straightjacket I have—it's easy to use with no terribly complicated parts. You could use me however you like." Len must have noticed my eyes widen in dismay. "Or we could just go out to dinner. I also think you'd like my cats."

"You have cats?" I was delighted, as I'd long believed good men love cats. "Do you play bridge?" Could Len be a great guy for me—one who loves to travel, keeps cats and says "yes, dear"?

"No bridge. But I must warn you, the ClubFEM ladies do gossip, meddle and micromanage. So it's best to keep mum about what happens outside club events."

I nodded, as if I understood. We then exchanged phone numbers and parted.

He called me at home the following evening. "The great thing about BDSM is how it enables me to make a deep connection with a mistress," Len explained after our perfunctory greetings. "You see, it fulfills some basic needs we all have. I am not jaded. I want to see you. And I would really enjoy serving you."

"How would you like to serve me?" I thought myself fairly naive about all this and demanded more specific information.

"I'd love to serve you tea."

Tea? How lovely, tasteful and civilized. This fellow was clearly no alcoholic. (Little did I then realize "tea service" is a major fetish among cross-dressing submissive men.) Just the night before, Len had complimented me on the black Japanese kimono I'd worn—reason enough to conjure up the image of an exotic ritual Japanese tea service. "How would you like to serve me tea? In what manner?"

"I love how women look in skirts. Sometimes I'll wear a maid's uniform when I serve. It's kind of funny and most ladies really like it. One mistress gave me the name Lenora and it stuck. Look, it's all bewildering when first starting out, but totally worth the effort. It's fascinating. Fun. Emotionally satisfying. I will help you, as I sense we may click in other ways, not just BDSM."

Was this the right sort of guy for me? I had wanted a submissive man and *voila*, there he was. But I lacked the perspective to determine whether Len was acceptable. After our chat, I noticed it was past 11 p.m., the time my three cats had their last feeding. They were 13-year-old litter mates with pure white coats and light blue eyes. One of them, Orchid, had one bright green eye and the other blue, a trait referred to as odd-eyed. Both Orchid's head and eyes were oversized, far larger than her brother's or sister's. Her recent stroke had given her the appearance of those kitschy, sad, big-eyed Pity Kitties from the seventies. I quickly fed Oedipuss and Pinky, then changed into a terrycloth robe for Orchid's care.

Orchid, who could move all her limbs but not stand, was always held in my lap for spoon feeding. She never fought me at bath time and ate heartily, as one who accepted her lot but was determined to live. As a show of gratitude, she would lick my fingers after a meal or bath. She knew she was loved and how I tried to help her.

Early the next morning I dished out food for my two healthy cats, then spoon fed, bathed and dried Orchid before the hour and a half trip to work. My friends thought I had a brutal commute but I was used to it. I'd take the subway from 23rd Street, then nearly 150 city blocks up to 175th Street. There I transferred to a jitney which crossed the George Washington Bridge and traveled across New Jersey's Route 4, where I toiled. Because half of the jitneys had rock hard molded plastic seats, which hurt me while sitting, I would wait for a bus having *asientos suaves* (Spanish for soft seats). My seat mates were primarily Hispanic, mostly Dominican household workers headed for Englewood Cliffs or Teaneck suburban households. I imagined this maid brigade both cleaned and performed childcare. Observing them, I often remembered Lulu from my childhood. I was reared down South in the fifties, when a maid who also looked after the little ones was a *mammy*, not nanny. Lulu was a plump Black woman who wore a kerchief on her head and worked from nine in the morning until seven at night, when the last dishes were washed. She would then go home to her family, continuing the same cleaning and childcare duties.

I could recall from over 50 years earlier asking Lulu how she ever managed. "You're here early in the morning until after dinner, then you go home and take care of your family. I just don't see how you do it!" I exclaimed one day, prodding her for an explanation.

"Lordy, *chile*," she drawled, drawing out her words dramatically, "That's the life of Lulu. That's the life of Lulu!"

Twenty years later, I was dating men who envisioned a family in the suburbs with a working wife and mother. These guys were invariably sizing me up for the position. With all the teeming, constant male attention I'd received, it was mainly about the next fellow taking me to the new trendy restaurant...and of course, what he was lacking. These men regarded me as more rebellious than nonconformist, a piss-poor candidate for the necessary compromises and sacrifices to be made as a wife and mother. "You're too independent," more than one complained. But for a woman who admittedly disliked children, craved foreign travel and was a hardcore experience-junkie, remaining single was my best, realistic choice.

I had noticed the hordes of hollow-eyed women in their thirties, forties and fifties pouring into Penn Station or Port Authority—they looked dog tired even before their work day began. I'd seen them dragging themselves out of Manhattan at the day's end with a look somewhere between purpose and panic, rushing to get home and pick up their kids, relieve childcare, shop for or prepare supper. I wondered how they did it all and knew theirs wasn't the life for me. I imagined it was a hard life, an upscale version of Lulu's lot.

I didn't get the suburban lifestyle but I sure got the suburban job. Beginning in 1980 I was employed by a group of softcore porn magazines in New York City, with offices located right across from Carnegie Hall. The workplace was comfortable and spacious, the hours breezy and duties easy. Benefits included a 401K plan, medical and dental insurance, five paid personal days, plus twenty paid vacation days. But in 1993 the magazine group's owner sold the porn titles to a New Jersey based company. I was fired, along with everyone I worked with; we were then re-hired the very next week by the new owners under very similar terms.

I had been schlepping out to Jersey for 18 years, assigned to an office above a carport with no working heat or air conditioning due to a pipe break within. Neither my employer nor my landlord would fix it (the cost, they claimed, was prohibitive). Every winter I would work in temperatures so frigid I wore long underwear, shearling boots and a down coat indoors. I'd write smutty copy while stomping my booted foot, just to keep the circulation going and avoid frostbite. It was impossible to plug in a space heater—such an appliance would overload the faulty electrical outlet in my office, blow a circuit and cause several nearby computers to crash. On a few occasions this had actually happened, whereupon the fearsome seventyish gentleman who owned the company would burst into my ice freezer of an office. His face would redden and his wiry white hair stand on end, as if he had stuck his finger in my faulty electrical outlet. When he screamed, I thought he could be heard on the island of Manhattan. In summer, I'd plug in a small fan, which offered little relief from the sweltering heat. Despite my entreaties, complaints and evidence of physical suffering, I was never moved from this employment hellhole. After nearly a decade, management fixed the outlet and brought in an electric heater. It helped warm my head and torso but had little effect on my cold feet. Although spring and fall brought pleasant weather, I worked in extreme temperatures for half the year.

It was a half step above the Life of Lulu.

TWO

A Pony Party Plus Public Play

I CROSSED THE PEDESTRIAN BRIDGE, ENTERED THE office, made morning coffee, then booted up my computer to peruse the ClubFEM New York City chapter website. Their next *fete* centered around pony play and invitees would be permitted to bring "pony tack." I hadn't a clue what that might be. Nevertheless, I contacted the head-mistress asking permission to attend, then read their party rules.

At the New York City ClubFEM parties, members agree to be in the female dominant and male submissive roles at all times, with no switching. Good, I thought—no irksome, macho doms. Male partygoers show they are available by attaching a purple ribbon to their collar; but this ribbon does not obligate those called the slave to engage in play without their consent. These guys are expected to exude an air of servitude and submissiveness—serving the women drink or food, addressing them as "mistress" or "ma'am," always treating them with utmost respect. There is a dress code, but only for men. Their choices are a formal tux, sissy service attire (often a maid's uniform), or the standard ClubFEM slave getup—only a black bow tie collar plus black jockstrap on your birthday suit.

I could even go just to socialize or observe: their site specified there was no requirement for either gender to actively engage in BDSM while attending events. With confidence and relief in equal measure, I eagerly anticipated attending their party. I was hardly reticent: for years I'd thrown myself into participatory sex journalism, reporting on seedy strip clubs, swing emporiums, nudist colonies and the like. I'd also produced a few porn films. But even though I was a sex business veteran, I'd always been sexually conservative, never having had sex with another woman, engaged in a threesome or in anal intercourse. Neither had I ever experienced the trauma of a serious sexually transmitted disease or an abortion. Even with exposure to so much varied and extreme sexuality through work, I lacked the urge to experiment outside my comfort zone. If I had this raging libido (and I didn't) I always had a delicate constitution. Even when I was in my twenties, I was so sensitive: introducing a new lover to my Miss Muffy would often later result in some variety of temporary kitty itch. As an older woman, I had observed the way female porn stars pushed their limits by accepting multiple phalluses or larger toys into every orifice. One current porn star bragged how she'd had her rectum stretched open with a rib spreader (referring to medical equipment used in open heart surgery or on cadavers). Sex stars now appeared to be more stuntwomen than the erotic actresses they'd been 30 years prior, in what is now called porn's Golden Age.

I was in my office and should have been working, but considered ClubFEM attendance vital towards understanding my submissive male *Leg Action* readership. I had deadlines, a workload, other magazines to edit. Among them was a teen-themed hardcore magazine which contained a few confessional stories. I turned my attention to "Co-Ed Confidential," a piece which needed a rewrite—my freelancer had turned in ten pages of beat off material with zero motivation for all the sex action.

I examined the photos selected to accompany the fictitious piece and began the duties I was paid to perform. Editing porn copy usually took suspension of disbelief to new levels.

The images were of a dark, bearded fellow having intercourse in every imaginable position with a milk-fed blonde of approximate college age. The copy, by a supposedly anonymous female, described balling a Middle Eastern exchange student. But why would she do that? I began to rewrite, making the girl a resentful only child of over-protective parents who wouldn't let her go away to college. Taking her courses near home, she rebels by defiling a religious, virginal Muslim. But the pictures were all of anal sex. How could Ali be a virgin? O.K., I'll make him not Ali but *Ari*, an Israeli exchange student and sexually experienced former fighter in the Israeli Army. What happens when she finds out after the anal sex he's Ari not Ali, a Jew not an Arab? Oh, they become lovers and annoy her Jesus freak parents. The end.

A regular feature was "Senior Superlatives: The Girl Most Likely To..." Each month I'd fill in the blanks with some tawdry tale. The upcoming issue had "The Girl Most Likely To Win The Science Fair By Experimenting With Her Pussy." My own high school Senior Superlative had been Most Talented, yet the career I'd made for myself was somewhere between underwhelming and repulsive. When I graduated from journalism school at age 19, if I had known over 3 decades of porn awaited me, I wouldn't have just hung up my robe, mortarboard and tassel, I would have hung myself.

Porn was, like a mud pit that abuts a hog trough, something I just fell into. In 1978, I was walking down Manhattan's Sixth Avenue and encountered my old boss from a trade magazine, where I'd been managing editor. The guy, then working for the *Swank* magazine group, asked if I'd write some fantasies for one of their many erotic publications. I sat at my clickety-clack typewriter, knocked out three fantasies of a thousand words each and mailed them in. The porn editor soon got in touch with me. "These fantasies are from a male point of view. I want *your* fantasies. *Female* fantasies."

I confessed I had no fantasies save for finding a wealthy man who'd treat me in the manner I wished to become accustomed. Because the many *Swank* owned titles were mainly filled with softcore pictorials, copy (specifically a regular column) was needed for balance. I proposed a sex advice column, where readers would write in questions for me to answer. When the editor countered I lacked the authority to give any advice, I convinced him that I *did*, if I'd write in the persona of a gynecologist.

Though the exact title of this sex advice column now escapes me, I remember assuming the character of a Russian doctor, Dr. Leon Twatski. I initially wrote both questions and answers. But as the column caught on, readers would contact Dr. Twatski about such problems as genital warts, secondary impotence or inability to orgasm. Many of these authentic letters concerned a variety of sexual kinks or fetishes. The correspondence, coming from men who sought information and understanding, was overwhelmingly sincere. None seemed to be in on the joke a certain Dr. Leon Twatski did not exist.

He was written as such a maniac, I wondered how anyone could trust a doctor who only briefly answered a question in the magazine, then launched into an erotic tale about one of his many nubile patients, whose legs were always spread (feet placed in gleaming silver stirrups which twirled) and were thrilled to be probed with any number of intrusive instruments. The vodka-swilling Dr. Twatski would often have sexual contact with his willing female patients, who were smitten by his old-world charm. The sordid (and often convoluted) stories he spun about his Soviet Union youth ever intrigued them.

Dr. Twatski led to other work. In 1980, I was holding down a job at a trade magazine but freelancing so much porn *Swank* offered to bring me on staff and double my current salary. Men's magazines like *High Society*, *Oui*, *Cheri*, *Gallery*, *Genesis* and *Velvet* were just some of *Swank's* New York City based competition. Way ahead of this pack were the major three—*Playboy*, *Penthouse* and *Hustler*. Big budget erotic films were happening, porn was chic and the adult entertainment business seemed to be a glamorous growth industry that would soon merge into mainstream movies.

Thirty years later, porn magazines were still alive but not at all well, with circulation numbers rapidly declining and publications falling off cliffs. For the past several decades, I'd had dates size up what I did for a living, then deem me as a future liability for a two-income marriage. "Porno magazines?" they'd laugh. "How can they survive porn at home on video cassette or cable television?" But many of these men's magazines *did* survive—even after video cassettes gave way to DVDs, and porn DVD sales collapsed with the advent of internet streaming video.

Leg Action is on its last legs, I thought, as I walked over to the ClubFEM Pony Party. I carried a vintage round yellow vinyl smiley bag containing the pony tack my inventive friend, Hugh*, had made me. He'd been excited just to learn about the event. "Ask your pony to tie this rope around his wienie," he'd insisted, while holding a tied up jumble of white shoelaces. "You'll be the center of attention."

"Maybe I don't want so much attention."

"Oh please, just look at the smaller knot. Ask your pony boy to put his cock inside the slipknot and tighten it." Hugh then gave me another shoelace rein tied with an even larger slipknot, this one for the testicles. "That's for when you want him to halt. Don't be afraid to pull hard—he'll like that. Yank the penis line right to lead him that way and pull the balls line back to stop him in his tracks. It's as simple as that."

"Are you sure?"

"Of course!" he replied confidently. Hugh was a divorced fellow around my own age with the mentality and persona of a much younger man. Although Hugh was hardly a sub, he was a handy, ever helpful free spirit. Though we'd been friends for decades, ours was not a romantic or sexual relationship.

I could easily walk to the gathering, which was held only a few blocks from where I lived. Headmistress Reina was in her usual frothy mood as she greeted me at the door, took my 20 dollar admission fee and handed me a leash. "You can attach this leash to any male with a purple ribbon on his collar," she advised, between giggles.

I was mindful of ClubFEM's rules concerning collared slaves without purple free-to-play ribbons, men who belonged to a certain dominant woman. Len had warned me how I couldn't even speak to such a fellow without his mistress's permission. I looked about the group of 20 submissive males and an equal number of dommes, happy to see everyone was over age 40 with the median age at about 50. Plenty of men were in their sixties with a few well into their seventies. In an aging crowd, I was still the oldest woman there.

But where was Len? As I searched the room, I imagined how I'd ride him. I then spied Len in a corner with a tall, tattooed mistress; she was holding him by a leash attached to a buckled leather open mask. It was hard to recognize him—in his open mouth was a ball gag nearly the size of a tennis ball. I doubted he'd seen me, as he wore wide blinkers on each side of his harnessed head. Len was garbed in a pair of leather pants but shirtless, with his arms pulled back from his torso and tightly wrapped in a leather device called an armbinder. I walked over and placed myself squarely before his tied-up face. "Hiya, Len!" I grinned.

Recognizing me, he issued a fairly credible whinny coupled with lowering his bound head. One of his feet pawed the sawdust-strewn floor. "He's in his horse space," his mistress explained, as she pulled on a leash, which drew him closer to her. He was obviously attached to this woman in other ways as well—I noticed there was no purple ribbon tied around his collar. He could possibly even be collared to this woman.

"May I pet your horse?" I addressed her only.

"Yes, you may. You're new here," she said, reading my name tag, "Mistress Pussycat." I stroked Len's balding head as he gave a little snort. "How do you know my sub?"

"He sat next to me at the last munch." As I left the lovers, I imagined leather blinders, harness and a ball gag would do little to keep him from straying outside his mistress's stable.

Reina and another guy in fancy dressage gear now began a joint lecture on pony play, while passing around fetish magazines like *Equus Erotica* and *The Human Horse*. Before the party, I'd studied online and was now familiar with images of men decked out in saddles, bridles, and bits. They carried women on their backs either piggyback style or on all fours.

The male lecturer wore a buckled leather harness around his torso and a fancy open leather mask with white plumes on top, as if his inspiration were the Lipizzaner show stallions from Vienna's Spanish Riding School. The object of pony play, he explained, was to see how equine the sub can get. There is to be no talking between horse and mistress, he declared, as speech impedes one from getting into his horse space. (Exactly what his mistress had been saying when I inspected Len.)

We women were now to choose and dress our horses. I waited for others to match up, then approached the last guy left, Timmy*. He appeared to be the youngest guy in the room, in his early forties. "Say, will you be my horse? I only weigh 112 pounds." Timmy lowered his head and neighed before we joined the other horses and riders sifting through a box of pony tack. Several mistresses were grabbing long Dynel ponytail hairpieces for their sub's black jock strap and attaching them in the back. Others found saddles, spurs and stirrups in the box. I left my horse, who'd grabbed a leather bridle with plastic bit, and retrieved the string set within my yellow vinyl smiley. "Put this loop around your penis," I told Timmy, with a bit of authority. "And now this one around your testicles." He did so and swiftly, before I mounted his back and rode him around the circle of 20 crawling, woman-bearing human horses.

"Mistress Pussycat!" gasped Headmistress Reina as I confidently tugged the flesh-attached shoelace reins to the right or left of Timmy's broad back. I was the only female there who had dressed her horse's male appendage and led him around in such fashion, Timmy neighing with each pull. After other mistresses took notice, one helpfully suggested I lead those reins into a circular metal bridle piece, and in that way control Timmy's genitals with tugs behind the head.

It's role play, it's a power exchange, I reminded myself, and all about the woman being in control. As for the guys, they loved being objectified—viewed as show horses, beasts of burden or beloved pets. One horse in the corner obviously needed discipline—he was getting his haunches whipped with a leather riding crop.

"Is your back O.K., Timmy?" I inquired with genuine concern, all the while pulling the meat puppet strings. He whinnied as a reply. "The bit we put in your mouth—is it uncomfortable?"

"But that's exactly the point!" replied my horse.

"No talking!" Headmistress Reina admonished. "They're horses!"

"Mine is Mister Ed, the talking horse," I shot back. The older crowd got the sixties television reference and laughed as I spontaneously sang a bit of the *Mister Ed* theme song. The headmistress wasn't even miffed a newbie would break the solemnity of the occasion. Those in charge were happy if everyone was having a good time.

I'd noticed a distinguished looking man, about ten years older than I, who sported a ponytail attached to his jock strap. He wore knee pads and had even brought leather stirrups. As he approached, the man asked, his eyes downward in the proper submissive style: "Won't you ride me, Mistress?" I again joined the circle, now atop this older guy in knee pads, Kenny*. "Dig the stirrups into my flesh to make me go!" my new horse whispered. Before I could ask if it would hurt, I realized once more that was just the point. I kicked his ribcage.

In a corner of the room, a silver-haired gent was on the floor, lying at the heels of a black leather-clad mistress seated on a chair. She was poking his various tender spots (including his testicles) with her leather riding crop, toying with the man. The plump, fiftyish mistress wore lace-up latex boots and the silver fox was licking her stiletto heels as if he were a bear ravaging a honey hive. Over and again, Silver Fox would rise, raptly sniff around the woman's legs and ample thighs (which never parted) but when he came close to her private parts, he'd be pushed back down by her riding crop. The mistress was in control the entire time, and the tantalized guy appeared to be in a trance. As I would learn, he was in his sub space.

I had checked out Silver Fox when he came in late to the event—he was handsome and wore an obviously expensive black leather jacket. If I had been at a trendy restaurant with my girlfriends, on seeing this guy enter they'd size him up and mutter to one another "heavy hitter," their term for moneyed men. "O.C." I would add, with a knowing look—the girls all knew my shorthand for organized crime. Outside of this arena, who would imagine this man as a kinkster Sisyphus prostrating himself before a pair of thunder thighs?

Clinging to Kenny's back made me use muscles I didn't even know I had. I wondered whether his knees hurt as much as my poor inner thighs. After I slid off him and before I left the party, we exchanged phone numbers.

"My upper legs are so sore," I confided when we spoke the next day.

"I feel as if I'd had too much sex."

"You know what's better than sex? Public play!"

"Really? Give me an example, Kenny. What have you done?"

Kenny's last mistress, Ava*, who'd recently moved back to Europe, had been a bold woman during her years stateside. Though Kenny lived in the suburbs, Manhattan had been their playground. For years he'd done whatever Mistress Ava required, often involving various public stunts meant to humiliate him. She once ordered Kenny to kneel on the Central Park lawn, where she blindfolded him and left him alone with a sign taped to his back. According to Kenny, several hours of kneeling passed, a length of time often punctuated with applause. Mistress Ava was observing her sub from a vantage point far away, noticing how passersby were responding to the sign she'd surreptitiously placed on Kenny's back: "Clap if you think I'm an idiot."

Kenny recounted how one caper began, with Ava spritzing the crotch of his pants with a water spray bottle, making him appear incontinent. She'd already instructed him to dress poorly. As Mistress Ava led Kenny down into the New York City subway system, she'd commanded: "Take off that stupid cap you're wearing, get down on your knees and beg for money. Keep an eye on me. When I touch my hair, I want you to sing 'God Bless America' and when I touch my nose you must give away all the money you'll have in your cap."

According to Kenny, he was quite the capable beggar. Riders filled his cap with coin as he crawled through the shuttling subway cars. A few hours into this profitable exercise, Kenny was confronted with some competition—a real beggar, obviously blind and severely disabled, entered the subway. After Kenny saw Ava touch her nose, he walked on his knees over to the blind man and emptied all coins and bills from his cap, giving it all away to another, just as his mistress had directed. She then touched her hair, signaling for Kenny to break into song. Shortly after he did so, the entire subway car joined in the patriotic tune, so moved were they to see one beggar giving an even more pathetic beggar all of his money. None suspected this interaction stemmed from the public play kink, and was acted out by a submissive man and his domme.

"You really ought to get into public play," Kenny suggested. His wife of 40 years knew all about Kenny's kinks. Laura* wasn't in the lifestyle herself, but received a regular earful about her husband's shenanigans. Kenny declared he and his wife were very close and he'd never cheated on her. "This isn't sex!" Kenny asserted. Then he asked, "Think you can come up with any public play as creative as Mistress Ava? Something really humiliating?"

I was up for the challenge. Kenny expressed only one caveat—no open displays of unusual sexuality. He emphasized people in the lifestyle went out of their way not to shock regular folks, the vanilla. "It's an imposition on others and we have to be respectful of their space."

"I feel limited," I groused during one of our many phone calls. "Look at groups like Improv Everywhere, who pull together hundreds of creative New Yorkers for stunts like their Frozen Grand Central. Think bystanders weren't freaked out seeing these IE agents carry out their mission by freezing in place?"

"But there was no sexual element to it," countered Kenny.

"How about every year when they do the Pants Off Subway Ride with all the chicks almost bare-assed in their bikini bottoms and the dudes wearing jockey shorts."

"You can do sexy. Just don't make it too obvious of a fetish thing."

Though it *is* a fetish, public play is not so different from performance art. Under the willing command of another, a player interacts with the public doing things (often embarrassing) he would not ordinarily do. On the surface, public play may seem like college hijinks or a hazing ritual; but in the context of BDSM, it is about humiliation and control.

It took me about two weeks to come up with a suitable stunt. Kenny and I met up near Penn Station; we'd later walk to our lunch destination. "I knew a woman who lived in that building." He casually pointed to a residential high-rise near Eighth Avenue. "She's into cutting. I had her cut a big initial letter into my back about ten years ago. It looked great while you could still see the scars, but before long it healed on up."

I almost stopped in mid-traffic. "Did you have any anesthesia?"

"Of course not—that would defeat the whole purpose."

"And the purpose would be, what?"

"To experience what it would be like. It was really interesting to feel the blade as it cut into the different layers of skin. Each offered a different pain sensation—the dermis different from the epidermis, and then..."

I interrupted him. "I'm going to have you do a challenge here." We'd come upon a tree-lined concrete pavement within a park-like setting. "Watch me carefully. Every time I place my hand on a tree, I want to see you make love to it."

I walked several paces ahead, before stopping to touch a tree growing fairly close to the sidewalk. Not even half a minute later, I turned around to see Kenny press his groin against the tree trunk, his outflung arms caressing its branches. I walked ahead and patted yet another tree. He sauntered up to it as if it were the most beautiful woman in a room filled with beautiful women. His tongue began to probe a knot conveniently located at head level. Kenny's amorous pantomime was funny stuff enough, but the reactions from onlookers made me collapse in giggle fits.

Kenny caught up to me after I'd sat on a park bench. "Time for a break," I laughed, shedding my sandals. Kenny got down on his knees without hesitation, immediately took one of my legs in his hands, placed a foot against his chest and began to massage my calves. At one point, he lifted my foot almost to his lips, coming close to licking the toes, but then put it down as if he thought better of it—we were in public. I could only sit on a hard park bench for scant minutes, so we soon arrived at Del Posto, which had the best luncheon *prix fixe* in town. It was an elegant place with superb service and, most important, a rest room well situated for our public play. Only a week before, I'd staked out their cushy can to examine whether their toilet paper was in squares or on a roll. Once I saw the roll, I made reservations and hatched a plan.

After a delightful multi-course lunch, I insisted we split the bill as Kenny was a friend, a married man and not my date or lover. As we savored the after-dessert petits fours and signed for the charges, I presented Kenny with a roll of tape and safety pin. "After they return our credit cards, visit the men's room—I want to see a long roll of toilet paper trailing behind you."

"Mistress, I can do that even without tape or pins," he assured in an efficient butler's voice. Kenny promptly left for the loo. Waiting for him at the table, I noticed Del Posto was still full. The bathroom was situated in the back, and to exit the restaurant he'd have to walk a center aisle visible to diners on both sides. Kenny and I hadn't made a much noticed entrance—but we would certainly make a dramatic exit.

I soon saw him leave the bathroom with six feet of ass-wipe coming out of his back waistband as he confidently loped towards the front door. Several patrons noticed this dapper gent trail the TP—a ghastly sight, especially with a waitress scurrying after him frantically calling, "Oh, sir. Oh, sir!" I scanned the diners' faces and found many amused, some agog, only a few oblivious to the scene. But the reaction I'll most remember was from the snooty *maitre d'*. Though his attitude when seating us had been fairly grand, as he witnessed Kenny's paper trail exit, his expression changed from one of boredom to a look of unabashed glee. He'd be dining out on this story for weeks to come.

When Kenny and I began walking the High Line back towards Penn Station, I was laughing so hard my mascara began to run. I used his toilet paper tail to wipe my eyes as we passed the Frank Gehry-designed IAC Building. Kenny had now completed all his challenges, felt totally empowered and wanted to share this feeling with his wife. He reached her on his cell phone. "I did it, baby! I did it! Mistress Pussycat really put me through my paces. You've got to meet her."

"Laura is dying to meet you, too," he whispered, while still on the phone.

Kenny often spoke of his strong marriage based on honesty and trust. I had no idea how that meshed with his more radical activities, in which his wife of 40 years refused to participate. "I tell Laura everything," he proudly confided.

"Even about the butterfly board?" Kenny was often present at lifestyle workshops and events. During lunch he'd reminisced about one lecture he'd demonstrated, on how to safely use a butterfly board. (This is a wooden tray which fits beneath a guy's equipment with the scrotum and penis dragged through. The testicular sac's thin outer skin is then pierced with needles and pinned to the board in several places.) No pain, endurance test or humiliation was too much for Kenny—it was always a challenge.

"Of course, the butterfly board," he responded. "And the saline injection."

"What's that?"

"It's when they inject a saline solution into your testicles. It makes them blow up to the size of a baseball, at the very least."

"You've got to be kidding. Why?"

"Mistress Pussycat, you need a basic BDSM education and I need a mistress to play with at the upcoming TES-Fest."

I conjured a mental image of a convention with a leather-clad, rope bound kinkster in every booth. Kenny promised if I joined him at the conference, he'd teach me everything I should know about BDSM in a single weekend. The Eulenspiegel Society (called TES) is a New York City based 39-year-old organization dedicated to the liberation and education of sexual minorities (with an emphasis on those practicing BDSM). The group sponsors frequent lectures, workshops, meetings, parties and addresses myriad sexual interests. Without the least bit of hesitation, I agreed to attend.

THREE

More Of A Pussycat, Less Than A Mistress

TES-FEST WAS HELD AT A WELL KNOWN HOTEL chain situated in one of New York City's many suburbs. Volunteers kept vigilant watch at all entrances and exits (to bar any vanilla) and issued all attendees special wristbands plus dog-tag IDs. As TES-Fest had reserved and taken over the entire hotel, the only vanilla about were some wide-eyed hotel staff plus two local cops paid overtime wages to survey their sweetest police beat ever. Because no outsiders intrude, none are shocked and no attendee's privacy is compromised.

Kenny handed me a schedule. We'd agreed to do TES-Fest together and had to choose the workshops we'd both attend. (There was much hands-on instruction which required a partner.) I tried to concentrate on the morning classes but became distracted by other attendees inside the hotel lobby. Several six foot tall guys who dressed in women's clothes wore makeup, glamorous wigs plus a beatific smile on their faces. They were blissed out to be liberated—finally in the open about their cross-dressing and among others accepting of them. This cathartic self-expression was found among leather folk, heavy chain wearers, people in bunny costumes and those decked out in horse gear.

The submissive women tended to rock black fishnet hose worn with high heels beneath short plaid kilts; above the waist it was more about piercings, multiple tattoos and eye-popping cleavage. Even though they were not exactly equal within their relationships, the percentage of male dominant to female dominant attendees was roughly equal. All kinky couples acted as if they were very much into each other—their mutual attraction appeared stronger than among the many married folk I knew who were not into the lifestyle.

"Come on, let's make a decision, the first workshop starts at ten!" Kenny urged.

There were seven choices on the schedule. "The course on Feral Play—what's that?"

"Biting and scratching. How about this lecture—Embarrass, Humiliate, Degrade and Objectify: Basics of Psychological Status Play."

"That sounds interesting. But what about the one called Sounds and Catheterization? I had a catheter put in at Johns Hopkins by a student nurse who didn't know what she was doing and it hurt like hell, since she tried several times. So, these sounds—are they going to play New Age music while they give some guy a catheter?"

Kenny shook his head. "Sounds are a device urologists use to correct obstructions in the urethra."

"And the point of this would be, what?"

"Pain. Pain and more pain, that's the name of the game. Interested in whipping? You could learn how with Single Tail Whips For Beginners."

"I used to like Zorro on TV but I'm not into whips. Hey, look at this course—Sufi-Inspired Strategies for Pain Processing."

"Now that really sounds New Age," countered Kenny. "Did you notice Techniques To Take Your Bondage To The Next Level?"

"I'm no good with ropes, Kenny. I can only tie the most basic knot; I'm not dexterous at all." We walked between the rooms, all rapidly filling.

We finally agreed on the lecture Components of a Submissive's Psychology, as it sounded fairly basic. It was led by a pleasant looking, well-spoken man in his mid-thirties who identified himself as a submissive. Of the dozens of workshops offered, half were on how to play, and the rest about the psychology and dynamics of BDSM relationships. Our lecture had a good deal of audience participation, so I could hear not only from femdom influenced pairs but from male-dominated couples. I had no idea why any woman would want to be in a relationship—with a man she called "Master"—where she was encouraged not to detach her own automobile seatbelt. Why would she get on her knees so Master could take off her collar before she showered? Yet these ladies professed to enjoy such protocols and rituals. As one explained, "It's all expressions of my role, a constant affirmation of my place as a submissive."

I was learning how the submissive's desire to please and perform acts of service sprung not out of masochism, but from a social and spiritual need. Our lecturer noted being submissive also gratifies when it's a release from being responsible, and remarked how many subs work at a high-pressure job all day. As it was explained: Top by day, bottom by night. (The words *top* and *bottom* were commonly used to represent *dominant* and *submissive.*) I remembered hearing similar sentiments from the kneeling fellows at DomSubFriends' speed dating event.

Our lecturer noted how in Buddhism, shedding the ego may lead to bliss and the submissive's arousal can be similarly spiritual. He also explained how the masochistic experience can often create powerful endorphins or could be purely erotic. Rules made by the dominant to the submissive (like no sitting on the furniture) can lead to sexual arousal when the sub experiences the humiliating act the dom or domme wants done (such as eating only on the floor). He called it "perving off on a lesser status."

"It's about getting your needs met." I nodded along with the rest of his audience. "If the top is into electrical play but the bottom only likes to be flogged—and the flogging holds no interest for the top, then your relationship is in trouble." There were even more understanding nods about the room but none from me. I wasn't looking to flog, but for a man who would say "yes, dear" or "anything you want." Was this a submissive man? For several decades, I'd been involved with so many males; but they were hardly seeking a woman just to make her happy. They wanted a live-in sexual satisfier who performed most of the drudge work in exchange for an even split of all expenses (regardless of income inequality). I called the many such proposals I'd received over the years "roommate situations." I wanted to be demanding, and become spoiled; but could I ever sell this to a submissive man as a compelling fetish? And would such a man satisfy me?

Before lunch, there was one more workshop to attend—Straight to the Point: Erotic and Intense Play Piercing. "If you have control of the needle, you have control of *her*," our middle aged female lecturer asserted. "Once the needles are in, it doesn't really hurt until you play with them." She demonstrated on a young woman who reminded me of the full-figured females found in Renaissance paintings. This compliant miss drew her breath in an audible hiss as each needle painfully pierced her creamy skin. I cringed while seeing her beautiful, sizable breasts being poked by several long ones, including some through her pinkish areola. She now began to pant and moan when even more long needles were driven under the skin of her ribcage, which the lecturer divulged was very sensitive, as were the inner thighs. Our demonstrator was then directed to spread her legs so thinner acupuncture needles could be placed on each side of her exposed vagina. The rapt audience watched as the girl squirmed.

Our instructor informed us there were two ways of taking them out: "The nice way and the not nice way." The latter was with the needle's bevel up, which not only hurt more but created internal bleeding. The lecture's end was met with appreciative applause, especially for the beautiful and bloodied young demonstrator. I left the room feeling a little queasy.

"The food at the hotel is kind of overpriced," Kenny complained as we filed out of the room. "Want to do lunch at a Chinese place nearby?"

"Jesus, Kenny, I don't know if I can eat right after seeing that."

"You'll get over it. Just put something in your stomach."

Of course he was right. I soon recovered, even before we'd ordered our combination plates at a local mall's Chinese joint. Kenny was calling his wife, Laura, telling her about the morning's lectures. I was on my cell phone to Marisa, Orchid's caretaker, finding out whether Orchid ate for her, if she'd wet her pad and had her bath. After attending TES-Fest, I'd determine whether Marisa could do everything necessary for Orchid's care—the feeding, bathing and tummy massage for defecation. If all went well, I would pay Marisa to do the same tasks in September, when I'd planned a two week vacation in Slovenia.

"Feeling better?" Kenny saw I was eating well.

"Much. Noodles have always been my comfort food."

"You can't let watching that stuff bother you. Not if you want to become a domme."

"I can be dominant without inflicting pain. Right?"

"Come on, you've never done anything even slightly sadistic?"

"Well, sometimes when I see a man in his fifties with his much younger wife, usually a second wife, and their small young'uns, I'll come up to them and say in my sweet Southern lady manner: 'What a good grandpa you are to those children!"

"You've never physically hurt a partner?"

"Not yet. But I've agreed to learn so..."

"So you'll join me in the dungeon tonight!"

"You can count on it."

Although Kenny identified himself as a submissive man, he was more of an experience junkie. There's an expression used in the BDSM community for guys who say they're submissive but control all the action and call the shots—they're "topping from the bottom." As I was hopelessly green (and now, sometimes a bit green around the gills) I was willing to let my submissive, Kenny, take the lead.

I perused the schedule with glee. "Look at this course, Massaging Masochists. Guess people want to learn how to give massages guaranteed to hurt. Hey, I'm too old for this lecture—Once a Month Menstrual Play. And probably this one, too—Squirting 101."

"You've got to learn CBT and this afternoon there's an introductory course in it."

"O.K. What's CBT?"

"Cock and ball torture."

"Why should I learn that? Is it a basic, one of the foundations of a domme's skill set?"

"Many submissive men like it. If you want to control a sub, you've got to learn CBT. And it's a skill you'll be using for the rest of your life," he noted, in the way I was told at age 13 the benefit of learning Latin.

Our instructor was a plump and plain middle aged nurse. One of her three male demonstrator volunteers (who all stood naked before the class) had a Prince Albert piercing—a little metal barbell going from the top of his penis straight through to the urethra. "Wait and have your kids before you have anything put in," our nurse-teacher advised. She further specified why she did not advocate any piercing of the testicles. "Permanent piercings present a long term tunnel of germs into the body, so you don't want to pierce an organ."

She began with what she termed a "simple whirlybird." As our instructor wrapped a length of small gauge rope around a demonstrator's penis, Kenny muttered, "This is fundamental CBT." Once the guy's penis was encased, like a kielbasa wrapped in an open grid pattern of plastic, our lecturer abruptly tugged the cord's end, which sent the guy's flaccid penis flying in every direction as he groaned aloud. It seemed jarring, to say the least.

"Don't tie up a man's balls when you hit them," she counseled. "But you can get a penis out of the way by tying a string around it and over his neck." She did just that, while explaining, "You can do some squeezing of the testicles—but not front to back, just side to side." I craned my neck to see over the others exactly what she was doing. Our instructor went on to beat her demonstrator's balls with cymbal whisks, weight loaded gloves and a dishwasher brush before pulling two paddles out of her bag. "You like these?" She confronted her sub.

"I thought this was supposed to be an introductory class," he groused.

"Don't worry," she replied, "I won't hurt you any more than you need."

"She's got a great attitude, doesn't she?" commented Kenny.

"Note how I'm paddling with the small side," she told her class. "And be careful of the testicular sac's upper area. When he's not erect, you can have more fun with it." She finally untied his penis, only to begin beating it with a ruler.

Next came the parachute, a small leather, conical-shaped collar fastened around our demonstrator's scrotum. Hung from the parachute were three short metal chains, to which our teacher attached various weights. The effect on the testicles was one of dragging and squeezing. She suggested lesser weights be added when a man is free to move, but heavier weights for when he is immobilized in bondage. Some 60 men and women were seated before her, many taking notes, as if planning to use these techniques in future scenes.

At the end of the hour lecture she warned: "Never hit a man in the back of his testicles while doing ball busting as it can cause permanent painful damage. And also, never wear buckled boots." The CBT workshop participants broke into appreciative applause for Nurse Nasty and her game demonstrators.

"What's ball busting?" I asked as I followed Kenny out of the room.

"When a woman kicks a guy in the nuts over and over again. Some guys love it."

We went to dinner at a Spanish joint and split a big dish of paella before using cell phones to call our loved ones. "I love you," Kenny cooed to wife Laura.

I had Marisa put the phone next to my blind cat's pink tinged ears. "I love you," I told Orchid over and again. "Did she poop for you after dinner?" When Marisa assured me she had, I was relieved. "Have you been watching *The Tudors* on Showtime?" Marisa didn't have premium cable channels at home as I did, so I'd recommended she watch this historical drama on my TV set.

Of course she had. "I've seen almost every episode of the last season, one after the other, for about eight hours today. God, those Englishmen were cruel, not to mention all the torture carried out during The Reformation. All about the different churches formed to worship Christ. Some of those scenes were so gruesome, I had to fast forward."

I'd had the same reaction. But I could not fast forward through the shrieks (all from women) I heard that evening after Kenny and I entered the hotel's ballroom-turned-dungeon. The two local policemen stationed there were chatting amiably with various members of the leather 'n studs crowd. With Kenny in tow, I toured the ballroom to see who was doing such impassioned screaming. Over in a corner, a man in his mid-thirties was flogging a woman approximately the same age. She was spreadeagled and bound to an X-shaped piece of equipment on which she writhed; her dramatic cries sounded as disturbing as anything I'd heard on *The Tudors*.

"She's on a St. Andrew's Cross," Kenny explained. "See, she's restrained at her ankles, wrists and waist." I asked him why they gave such a devilish thing the name of a saint. "It's the same diagonal cross shape St. Andrew was martyred on."

"Look, the policemen over there seem totally unconcerned." I gestured in their direction.

"They know he's not really hurting her that much. She's getting off on being flogged and he's perving off on her vocals. It's consensual. They're in a scene." Kenny imagined they were a married couple who would do this in their basement, were it not for the kids around the house. "This is their escape from suburbia."

There were more howls coming from a blanket nearby—a woman was having a man pour hot candle wax on her chest and midriff. Kenny explained: "Look how he drips the wax from an exact point high above her. He's giving the wax time to cool before it hits. Now if he were flinging the wax from a candle just a few inches away, her screams would be real."

With some sort of sadomasochistic activity was going on every few feet, the ballroom was packed with kinksters, often using various bondage equipment. I noticed a beautiful young thing who was having an older woman wrap a long blue ribbon shoelace-style on her nude torso. It appeared as if strawberry jam had been slathered about, making a vivid blue and scarlet palette on the girl's pale flesh canvas. "Is that food play over there?" I glanced in their direction.

"You're talking about the multiple piercing over there? She's getting laces put on all the needles she's had inserted."

"Oh, that's blood?" My attention now turned to an attractive, young naked guy in his twenties. He was tied to a T-shaped wooden post which had almost a crucifix look about it. Two pretty girls took turns backing up, taking aim and kicking him in the testicles with the tips of their bare feet. The fellow would noticeably flinch in pain after every blow, only to recover and after a minute or so have the other girl kick him in the crotch once again.

I grabbed Kenny's arm. "Are they doing the ball busting mentioned in CBT class?"

"That's it. Watch the precision of those girls' feet when they strike. They hit it in the front. It may hurt, but no one gets hurt." (This nut crunching scenario continued for several minutes before the two girls untied the young guy and all collapsed into a three way hug.) "These girls know what they're doing and have obviously done it before. Now *you've* got to get some experience. What are you going to do to *me*?" Kenny radiated an air of anticipation.

As I led him towards the middle of the room, I demanded he give me a massage. There was an empty table. I was the domme and I called the shots. This was what I desired and my sub had to comply. As I hopped up on the table, Kenny put the big duffle bag he carried beside it. I kept on my cotton sundress as he expertly administered a full body massage. My moans of pleasure soon joined the assorted cries and whimpers about the hotel ballroom-turned-dungeon. It was like being at a spa in the midst of Dante's Inferno. There was no penetrative sex being performed on the premises, and certainly none of the extreme acts which had dominated the adult film business for the past two decades. The *bukkake* films (where women are covered in semen by dozens of men at once), the gang bang flicks (where one female takes on a hundred men) and all the multi-phallus action (more concerned with stretching and stuffing than satisfying) had long become standard erotic fare for vanilla men.

As my muscles relaxed with Kenny's massage, I compared what I'd seen at TES-Fest to the porn flicks American teenagers often consider their sex education. What went on in the dungeon seemed very personal, as opposed to typical over-the-top and incredibly impersonal vanilla porn action. Girls on porn sets would never even be there or consider performing such acts, were they not earning several hundred dollars for their scene. And porn stars had no say in choosing their on-camera sex partner (unless they were among the few chosen elite contract girls). I'd been on enough sets to witness how erotic entertainers often looked bored or unhappy off-camera. By comparison, the shrieking suburban dungeon dolls wanted to be there, do more or less what they were doing, and probably with that exact person.

After about 20 minutes of being alternately kneaded and caressed, I began to detect pressure of a more familiar sort—Kenny wanted action. Or rather, he wanted to be hurt with an urgency that reminded me of past lovers, and how their needs had led me to intercourse. "Let's do The Clouds," he suggested for about the fifth time, mentioning how they have this at every TES-Fest.

If we did The Clouds, we'd have to miss the slave auction, where attendees bid for a session with some of the better known workshop teachers. It was all for a good cause, The National Coalition For Sexual Freedom. This organization upholds the civil rights of those facing discrimination for expressing any unusual sexuality. Employment (and other) discrimination against homosexuals is against the law; but heterosexuals who cross-dress, openly engage in bondage and domination, are obviously into swinging or a leather lifestyle have no such law protecting them. NCSF is a civil rights organization, but for kinksters.

Cloud Nine and Cloud Ten were two sizable hotel room suites physically near each other, but they served two separate functions. After entering Cloud Nine, volunteers gave Kenny and I a choice of cider or sweet tea. We could keep our clothes on or change into terry cloth robes. Hypnotic New Age music played in the background and a familiar incense filled my nostrils. I chucked off my sun dress for their robe before the unfazed Kenny, who had seen much nudity through the years. In a soothing mode, my volunteer masseuse inquired whether I had pain, where it hurt, and how I liked to be touched during massage. It was one of the best 30 minute therapeutic massages I'd ever received and free of charge. Kenny received a similar treatment in the adjoining room.

We were both loose and relaxed when we regrouped. "Now it's time for Cloud Ten!" he exclaimed. As we entered the room, loud, driving acid rock music mixed with the grunts and groans of an unseen couple having intercourse. As a stab at privacy, sheets had been taken off beds and used as makeshift partitions. A bowl of wrapped condoms sat on a nearby table.

Kenny put his duffle bag near the bed, and from it retrieved a length of small gauge rope. "You saw the whirlybird demonstrated in CBT class," he began in an assured voice. He unzipped his fly, yanked down his pants and sat on the unmade hotel bed. "Why don't you practice your technique?" Kenny had his flaccid penis in his palm—his other hand held the rope for me to manipulate.

"Tell me if I'm not doing this right," I begged as I took his manhood in hand. Kenny was now lying on the bed, rope wound around his penis, waiting for me to firmly yank its tail. I pulled the end quickly, the way I'd seen old lawnmowers started, then watched as his penis was roughly jerked around. An audible deep moan from Kenny became nearly drowned out by a much louder orgasm from the man two sheets over, in our same space. "Didn't that hurt?" I asked him.

"Of course. But it's hard to screw up a whirlybird, it takes zero skill. Let's see your knife play technique."

Knife play? I had yet to see this demonstrated—images of magicians throwing daggers at their scantily clad female assistants sprang to mind. Kenny rummaged through his huge bag until he found a large knife. "Here, trace it around my entire genital area. But be sure you use the tip of the blade and not the edge." He unsheathed the knife and handed it to me. As long as my spread hand, it had a curved blade end and mother-of-pearl handle. Kenny lay back down to anticipate his next sensation. With trepidation, I slowly and lightly circled his penis and testicles with the knife tip.

As I inched the blade towards his jewels, I heard his dramatic, sibilant intake of breath. "Kenny, am I hurting you?" The couple next to us had calmed down.

"No. Just keep doing it and don't spoil the mood."

After three slow circles, I put down the knife and barked, "Next!"

"Ever see a Humbler?"

"One of those big German cars?"

"Not a Hummer, a *Humbler*." Kenny sprang up from the bed, placed the knife back in his bag and came up with yet another kinky appliance. "This is no ordinary Humbler—I hand carved, polished and lacquered it myself," he proudly noted, before pulling a felt bag (the kind used to cover fine silver) off of a two-foot long, wing-shaped device.

"Lovely grain on the wood there," I pointed out, in the way of a compliment. The thing had two separate bars which, when fastened, formed a notched hole in its middle.

"It takes a while to get the hang of it, so let me show you how this works." Kenny unlocked the device, wrested its two bars apart, then bent his knees while taking both his testicles in one hand. He then pulled all of his genitals back and through his legs before clamping the Humbler in place. Now bent at the waist, he turned around to display a bare butt with his penis and scrotum centered beneath and emerging from the long wooden contraption.

"And the point of this is, what?" Kenny lurched and hobbled about the now empty Cloud Ten. Despite the fact his package was coming out of his ass, he was having a grand old time—the man was having a ball with his balls.

"The Humbler is a physical restraint and once it's on, you can't straighten your legs without painfully pulling on your testicular sac. See?" Kenny's moves reminded me of Groucho Marx's bent walk—all he needed was a cigar to flick. He now pointed out the several wooden clothespins he'd placed on his duffle bag handles. "Take one of the smaller ones and put it on my nipple," he whispered.

Kenny closed his eyes and winced as the clothespin pinched. "Both nipples," he murmured.

"O.K., just let me know if it hurts too much."

"A domme never says anything like that," he groaned while I placed the clothespins. "They just ask the sub for their safe word—not as if *I* need one." He suggested I strike the clothespins with the side of my hand. As I did so, Kenny threw back his head dramatically; his aging features assumed the visage of a suffering saint.

The clothespins now off, Kenny was still eager for more. "You've got to learn how to trample." He sprang from the bed to lie face up on the carpet. "First thing to remember: never wear high heels or you could puncture a lung. Actually, you should only trample barefoot. Now, walk on my torso but don't put all your weight on my middle. Instead, place your feet around the edges."

"You're too thin!" I tried to follow his instructions without losing my balance.

"O.K. Just keep one foot on the floor. Use the other to lightly kick my cock and balls."

Some submissive man, calling all the shots, I thought, as my toes made contact with his nuts. But I was learning how to be a dominant and Kenny had offered some hands-on practice sessions. And he'd never intimated any sex was involved. Getting off with hand jobs, blow jobs or intercourse wasn't his thing—he was into being hurt.

"Get up, Kenny, or I'll miss my train back to the city." I hadn't planned on staying over and it was getting late.

He slowly rearranged his lanky form into an upright position. "Your luggage is checked at the front desk, right? Why don't you come home with me tonight and sleep in our guest room. I think you and my wife would really hit it off. Then we can take more workshops tomorrow. I'll call Laura and let her know."

"All right, Kenny. I just have to get in touch with my cat sitter."

"And then we can bathe in the hotel's hot tub, it's very therapeutic."

"Oh, that sounds great!" A jacuzzi was more my style. We were all alone in Cloud Ten; others were mainly interested in doing the dungeon, the see and be seen place.

"But you should practice your paddling before we leave." We'd earlier participated in Spanking 101. Kenny reached into his bag, grabbed a paddle, and motioned for me to sit bedside. He handed me the paddle before draping his bare body over my knees. "Aim for the sweet spot." This would be the lower buttocks on a guy but higher on a woman, I'd recently learned.

"Harder! Harder!" Kenny urged with each successive whack of the half dozen I delivered. He then lifted himself up and mumbled, "I'm pulling out a thicker paddle. You have no strength." He rooted in his duffle bag and came up with a more substantial model. "Here, use this!" He arranged his body differently and waited for more blows. Again my strength proved insufficient, even as I tried swinging from the shoulders while keeping my wrists straight. I felt inadequate, not powerful or superior, and the entire exercise left an impression not of BDSM, but more like tennis lessons.

"I can barely feel that," Kenny complained after about a dozen hits from the half-inch thick wooden paddle.

"I'm going to call you Titanium Tushie," I teased, as he unearthed yet another instrument of pain from his long, Bad Bag.

"You have to use the cane. I don't pull it out for many people—but you're so weak."

"Kenny, your cheeks are already flushed beetroot. Isn't caning something they do in Singapore if you're caught spitting chewing gum on the street?"

"Caning is a fundamental. Now aim for the buttocks." Were it not for the crack in his ass, I could barely tell where his buttocks ended and upper thighs began. I took aim and finally he was now feeling the pain. "Keep going," he panted, after I'd landed a few hits with the thin, stinging cane. "I want to soak these fresh welts in the hot tub." And he wants others to see the marks I'd made, I concluded, while administering the final blows.

"Now *that* hurt." Kenny grinned while pulling on his pants.

"I have to stop by the front desk to take some swimwear out of my checked luggage."

"No one wears a swimsuit in the hot tub."

"Maybe not at home in the suburbs, but we're at a hotel."

"We're at a BDSM convention in a hotel. Say, let's go by the hot tub and if we see even one on anyone of either sex, I'll go with you to get your bathing suit."

"Deal." Walking through the lobby, we each made our calls—to cat sitter and wife—and soon approached the hot tub. After observing two heterosexual couples frolicking in the altogether, I doffed my dress and submerged myself in the warm, bubbling water. Kenny joined me and almost immediately struck up a conversation with one of the guys, right after his lady friend left the tub. From what I could gather, they resided in the submissive girlfriend's house.

This dominant male began to speak about his preferred web site, *Hog Tied*. "It's got all these girls who are bound with their backs, hands, feet together, so their vaginas are exposed and they're brought to orgasm again and again with all these wild toys. See, they have no control over any of the action. It's all forced orgasm—which is for me, a real turn on," he enthused. "My very favorite site," he declared, as though sharing with us his preferred tune or vacation spot.

"Let's go, Kenny!" I declared in a decisive tone as I lifted myself out of the hot tub. When I toweled off, he soon followed.

"Did that dom I was talking to bug you?" asked Kenny as he took my checked luggage.

"I find him and others of his ilk revolting." I guided my small wheeled suitcase toward Kenny's car.

"Now I think you *are* a domme," Kenny chuckled. "Some dommes simply despise dominant men. Say, you know what they call a dominant man who has lost his submissive lady?"

"No, haven't a clue."

"Homeless!" Kenny cackled. "It's an old joke in the scene."

"If it's funny, I don't get it. Explain, please." We drove out of the hotel parking lot.

"It's like this. You see a lot of dominant men who've found these women living alone, or alone with their kids. She's got the house from a divorce or something. The guys seduce the woman, then move in and totally control them. And if it weren't for this woman, that dom would have no life, not to mention nowhere to live."

"Is this also true for dominant women? Do they find submissive men who are more stable than they, before moving in with and controlling them?"

"No, not at all. The dommes are more independent and also less predatory."

"But all this talk of dommes having slaves. What's that all about?"

"Slaves are a whole other thing. We're talking about submissives here. Dommes want to see subs who can be of service. They like their subs to have certain skills. Dommes have their housecleaning sub, their handyman sub, their computer sub. And if they live in the city and have no auto, then there's also a car guy sub."

"Are they ever monogamous with a sub?"

"Only if they're collared or legally married and it's what was agreed on. Lifestyle dommes basically have submissive men in their life to please and serve them. But living off these guys as the masters do with the submissive women? That's rarely done."

As we reached Kenny's large, comfortable suburban residence, his wife, an attractive, petite woman in her mid-sixties, graciously welcomed me into her home. Laura related to me as though I were her husband's relative or business associate.

"I've been giving my Mistress some more hands-on experience." Kenny confided in his wife.

"I practiced my whirlybird technique." I offered.

"Oh, the whirlybird," she repeated, rolling her eyeballs with wry amusement at her adventurous spouse. Laura knew what I was speaking of, yet didn't seem to mind another woman's hands on her husband's dick. She shot Kenny an indulgent smile close to a smirk, as if she had his number and this was nothing she hadn't heard before.

"I got caned tonight. I've still got the welts," Kenny told his wife.

We soon all said our goodnights. It was past midnight, time to wash up and go straight to bed. Theirs was a marriage built on trust—Kenny shared all aspects of his life with his spouse. He didn't go on the prowl for sex outside the marriage, only sensation.

The next morning, their lively laughter and chatter greeted me before I entered the kitchen. Kenny stood behind his wife, who was at the sink, with his arms around her, dry humping as he reached around to squeeze a breast. He was obviously still interested in sex and theirs was not a dead marriage. Kenny was never touchy-feely or sexual with me. He did no flirting or romanticizing–he was just showing me the ropes, as promised. Kinky Kenny impressed me as a faithful married man.

The three of us spoke about travel during breakfast until it was time to leave. I thanked the serene, secure Laura for her hospitality before Kenny and I headed back to the conference. Driving there, we bickered about which afternoon class to attend–Bloodsports 201, Strap-On Basics For Any Hole, or Suspension.

I'd already signed up and paid for the Dominant Woman's Sunday Afternoon Tea Party. There Kenny would be serving as a butler–he'd already placed his tuxedo and dress shoes in his car's trunk. The tea ritual is big among submissive men who serve dressed as either as a maid, a sissy maid, or in formal attire (tuxedo). I'd seen plenty of sissy maids attending TES-Fest; these were bisexual or heterosexual men who cross-dressed as a servile woman.

The day before, I'd encountered Sissy Maid Stephanie, who ran a sissy maid academy. (Men pay to be trained as ladies-in-waiting while staying at a country retreat.) He'd shown me his fur-covered glove, and the five metal can opener tabs attached to it. "Just like a cat's paw," he purred, stroking and scratching my arm. A good sissy maid will do more than pour tea–he will draw a lady's bath, brush her hair, apply makeup, iron delicate lingerie. A sissy maid is gratified with anything bringing him closer to the feminine–even performing mundane household tasks–if it's at the command of a dominant woman. Sissy maids are not homosexual; they just identify with and express themselves by femininity.

The formidable Sissy Maid Stephanie was overseeing the Dominant Woman's Tea, riding his sissy maid staff hard, ensuring every detail would be perfect. Outside the Stephanie persona, he was a burly, bossy fellow in his mid-fifties with an outgoing persona and booming voice. As a sissy maid, he wore full makeup, a blonde wig and French maid's outfit accessorized with black fishnet hose and heels. Sissy Maid Stephanie didn't dress that way just to serve—I had seen him similarly garbed on the streets of New York, while fully exposed and uncovered by any coat. (Just in case any observers failed to get the point, *Sissy Maid Stephanie* was prominently embroidered in pink on his frilly black skirt.)

The sissy maids wore ruffled short skirts with several layers of stiff, starched crinolines underneath. Some sported ruffled white or pastel panties. Others wore no undergarments but had a little bell (the kind you see on pets) tied with a string attached to their penis. This ding-a-ling could clearly be viewed from the seated dommes' sight lines. When a domme summoned a sissy maid, one of them would scurry over—cock tinkling, mascaraed eyes twinkling, patent leather shoes gleaming, tea-pot steaming. These fellows were in a state of bliss, just to be serving and showing off this hidden side of themselves. Half of the dozen sissy maids wore traditional white-trimmed on black maid's outfits—the rest wore frocks made from juvenile themed, cartoon patterned fabric with clown-like wigs and makeup. These men found expression and satisfaction in their unique, bizarre appearance as if they were channeling the late, great Divine, star of many John Waters' films. The tuxedo-clad Kenny was the only guy serving tea, muffins and scones dressed as a male butler.

The dominant women were seated at four large tables, alongside anyone else who'd paid 40 bucks for a Sissy Maid Tea ticket. Though there were primarily dommes at my table of ten, a fiftyish dom and his ten years younger submissive lady were also seated among us. "I had the impression this event was only for dominant *women*," I bitched to an older domme who sat next to me, as the sissy maids poured. The dominant male couple certainly added a different perspective to our table conversation. The forty-something submissive brunette had been recently divorced and admitted she'd felt lost until she found "my dark Lord." He was a vegetarian so she'd abandoned all meat—except, perhaps for m'lord's staff—and currently cooked what and how he preferred. His long hair spilled over a black Aerosmith t-shirt. The year before, this relic from the Heavy Metal Era had uprooted himself from the New York City metropolitan area to live in Pennsylvania's mountains with his submissive sweetheart. He gave the dominant women at our table his very own recipe for a happy relationship: "It's just a lot of honesty and whole lot of sex."

The domme seated next to me, who was probably in her late sixties, asked him how long they'd been together. It had been six months since they met, he answered.

"It's always a lot of sex in the beginning," expressed the domme in a low, hushed voice only I could hear.

"Honesty from a woman is the last thing a guy like that can handle," I whispered back.

Since Master Metal had relocated to be with his ladylove, I grilled him about how he made his living. (He was at least a decade younger than the usual retirement age.) He confided he was doing the same thing as before moving in with his submissive—nothing more than living his life.

"You'd be surprised by how many dominant men who've found submissive women to live with are *in transition*," the wise domme tactfully explained. I remembered Kenny's joke about how a dominant man who had lost his submissive was called homeless, and began to see the kernel of truth behind the humor.

Once the tea was over, Kenny changed out of his tuxedo. As he drove me to the train station, I recounted what I'd observed about the dom.

"If lot of dommes really don't like dominant guys, that doesn't mean they can't love submissive men. You just have to meet more subs, see some action," Kenny noted.

"I never thought I'd be into hurting or humiliating a guy. I just want to call the shots and get spoiled. But now, maybe so, since I'm seeking a submissive man."

"But for getting where you want to be, you must develop your BDSM skill set. Pain is what these guys are seeking. As for humiliation, remember what you learned?"

"Humiliation is making someone do what they really, secretly want to do," responded his 60-year-old student. "But how do I find some guys to practice on?"

"Are you registered on FetLife?" Kenny drove into the train station. "It's a website for people in the lifestyle. The subs you want wouldn't come to a conference like this. They're all closeted, but probably online. You'll find plenty of action there and many choices for whatever it is you're looking for."

"I'm looking for something different—and lots of choices has always appealed to me." I thanked the kindly Kenny for giving me a memorable weekend and registered on FetLife the very next morning.

FOUR

My Passive Pantydropper

THE ONLINE AGGREGATOR, FETLIFE, WAS A GATEWAY to any number of websites where kinksters could connect, many searchable by sexual orientation, age and geographic area. I was only interested in meeting single submissive males—women, dominant men, married men and bisexual guys were out of the question. I also avoided those who identified themselves as *switches*—I had no intention of starting up with a sub, only to find how, on odd days, he turned into a whip wielding dom.

I drafted a rough idea of who I was (a Southerner living in Manhattan, one used to a sophisticated lifestyle) and what I sought (a chivalrous, submissive older man). My posting further specified:

> *No married men or men in long term relationships—you can only serve one mistress. If you are responsible for small children, or have joint custody do not reply. No bitches, no switches. And if you're bi...it's bye!*

I posted a picture that was 3 years old and subtracted 20 years from my age. When lying about my advanced years, I didn't feel even the tiniest pang of guilt. What then was the point of all the expensive plastic surgery I'd had, if not to allow me a few more years of feeling desirable and in control?

I anticipated few replies and wasn't prepared for the deluge of men who positively responded to my princess-like, demanding attitude. After receiving over 50 messages the very next day, I began humming the sixties Jan & Dean tune, "Surf City." This was Surf City in reverse, and way more than two guys for every girl. Most messages I received were well composed, using correct grammar and an expansive vocabulary, as if sent by thoughtful, intelligent men. The sender always used proper BDSM scene punctuation—lower cases when referring to themselves, and upper case letters for the dominant. After I replied to a sub, and we got a little dialogue going, they offered their cell phone numbers almost immediately.

"Are you single?" I asked a sixtyish prospect from New Jersey.

"Yes, lady, single with no living relatives. So if you keep me, I can be your property and no one will come looking for me. I'd be yours to use and abuse for as long as you like." His voice was even and measured, as if he were explaining the virtues of some appliance.

"Oh, I don't need a guy to be *that* single," I back peddled. "I just try to avoid married men. So, you live in the New Jersey suburbs, right?"

"Yes, but I would relocate anywhere, really. I love doing chores and I'm eager to learn, easy to train."

"It's good you don't seem so set in your ways."

"Very true, lady. I'm low maintenance and can live off scraps from your table. And I've no limits. I'd actually prefer a strict owner."

I had three cats, enough ownership for me. The Jersey boy was tame compared to the dark desires of Mr. Long Island, a man in his mid-fifties who'd stated he was single and interested in fine dining. I imagined I was becoming knowledgeable about the lifestyle when I queried him how he wanted to be regarded, as a *sub* or a *slave.*

"I would like to be treated as a *toilet* slave," he calmly responded.

"Oh, you're into the golden showers."

"Not at all!" He was a bit indignant. "I'm into discipline and behavior modification."

"But to what end? What does this accomplish?"

"I want to be trained to worship my mistress's waste so I can only orgasm with her feces in my mouth," he explained in a matter-of-fact manner. "I'd begin with a very small amount, force fed to me under restraint. It would be slowly increased to a full bowel movement." Rather than appear as a man with poor judgment, he quickly added: "But no more than one a week, for health reasons."

I still didn't get the point of this exercise in excrement and told him as much.

"The purpose is to eventually get an erection at the sight and smell of my mistress's feces. But I can only be in your captivity on weekends."

"Big job, right?"

"Yes, that plus a live-in vanilla girlfriend who has no idea what I really like."

Mr. Long Island sent me a link to his secret blog, detailing sporadic Saturday to Sunday exploits which would have offended the Marquis de Sade. As for the girlfriend, I wondered how he explained his weekend whereabouts—a fishing trip, perhaps? After he first contacted me, I initially thought he had money and thought he could take me to some choice restaurants. But that was before I learned his fetishistic fantasy eating preferences. My expectations needed to be more reasonably managed here.

One man from Connecticut asserted his ideal domme can be of any size, age or background. Anyone who accepts being dominated by an older woman piques my interest. Mr. Connecticut didn't play hard to get at the beginning of our phone chat. "Own me please! Let's make a life together! I'm ready to do anything to please you—just give me the chance!" His desperation repelled me and I soon ended the call. But I was too inexperienced to know how begging is a common fetish among submissive men. In reality, this fellow could possibly have had his pick of women—the begging act simply pushed his buttons.

Another liberal prospect affirmed he could be with any race or nationality, yet willfully disregarded Lincoln's Emancipation Proclamation. "You're Southern but you sound *white*. Oh, no, that won't do," he fretted. "I need a permanent no way out and no hope of escape real life slavery to a big Black woman." On learning I was as thin as I was white, he was disinterested in continuing our conversation.

Other men were similarly selective about who they'd serve and the life they'd lead. A fiftyish Floridian asserted he had contacted me because I resided in Manhattan. Mr. Florida didn't seem submissive in the least. In fact, he bombarded me with a series of questions, all to determine my wealth and social status. When he soon learned I was a middle-aged, middle-class ordinary employee, having received only a four-year degree from a state college, he asked whether I knew his sort of woman. "My lady is independently wealthy and very powerful in her vanilla life. She's highborn, accustomed to being catered to and doesn't need a man for money. A woman with brains is a real turn on—but if she looks like a supermodel too, all the better. If you could find me someone like that, even if you don't run in those circles, I'd like to become such a lady's slave husband." He then admonished me: "But forget introducing me to any who don't meet my standards. I won't submit to just anyone!"

Though I had a few girlfriends with money, none were powerful, and all would double up in laughter at the prospect of a *slave husband*. Mr. Florida was using his BDSM contacts as a means of achieving hypergamy, or marrying up. Unlike the many others who identified as slaves, he wasn't really aiming for a service situation.

Maybe I was seeking something that just doesn't exist—a normal submissive guy. As I entered a local munch, one where dominant women could meet submissive men, I wondered whether I still sported the same old shit-magnet that had stuck to me for the past few decades. Entering the diner's back room, I noticed there were twice as many seated men as women and chose a cushioned seat. It was directly across the Formica tabletop from a fellow who introduced himself as Mister Slave*. Peering over my plastic-laminated diner menu of overpriced fare, I observed a good looking man as hairless as Yul Brenner, Kojak or Mr. Clean. I also noticed many hair follicles all about his scalp: he was not naturally bald as much as consciously clean shaven. Mister Slave could have possibly had thinning locks, but he was hair free by choice.

"Mistress Pussycat," he chuckled, reading my name tag. "New here, huh? So are you a mistress or just a pussycat?"

"I'm a newbie lifestyle domme with three cats at home and I'm their mistress."

"I've kept cats, on and off, for most of my life. And I believe I'd be a good slave to a woman just beginning to explore her dominant nature." As there was plenty of chat going back and forth, up and down our table, I hadn't much opportunity to suss out this Mister Slave. From what I could gather, he aimed to worship and serve his one mistress, obeying all her rules. Compared to many subs, who I imagined purposefully went from one domme to the next, pleasing each and all, this Mister Slave appeared to prefer monogamy.

After dinner, I suggested we have a drink at Pars, my neighborhood's Persian joint, which was within easy walking distance. Although he was in his mid-forties and way too young for me, I blithely ignored the fact. I instead approved how he was tall, fashionably dressed and oozed sex appeal. After the recent TES-Fest weekend with Kenny, I was eager to go out on my own, using my new skills and dominant mindset on an exciting new guy.

Pars got a mixed crowd of Iranians lolling about on pillows alongside leather-clad kinksters who congregated around the bar, knocking back a few brewskis before trekking across the street to Paddles. On some nights, a belly dancer would take up the center of the room and there shake her ample hips. Every evening strangely forceful Middle Eastern music competed with the bar side TV, usually tuned to the Al Jazeera channel. "Don't you love this place? And it's right across the street from Paddles."

"So, you've been to Paddles," grinned Mister Slave as he leaned against the bar.

"Oh, sure—I live a few blocks away. Is Paddles your home away from home?" I had to know whether this self-assured guy was into the play-for-pain scene.

"I've been a few times. But I've never been into dungeons as a diversion or pastime. I don't go to pro-dommes. Never have, never will.

Don't need lots of major masochistic action. To create an overall erotic experience, there has to be some sort of attachment between me and my mistress. Sex? Well, it may or may not take place."

"You've never been spanked or paddled?"

"Of course I have. See, part of the deal would be submitting to my mistress's desires, even if they have an element of cruelty. If it is for *her* erotic pleasure that I submit, not mine. My mistress is always free to employ corporal punishment as she pleases. If she believes I need any maltreatment...then I just grit my teeth and bear it."

As we drank our wine (we were both big grape nuts) I inquired about his job. Mr. Slave worked long hours as a manager in the entertainment field. When he, in turn, questioned what I did, I divulged how I worked in adult entertainment.

"I'm impressed," he replied. "Shows me you're comfortable with your sexuality, that you're adventurous and can hold your own in a dominant fashion."

"Oh, I've never been in front of the camera. I'm on the editorial side."

"So, you've been across the street. What'd you do there?" His manner was off-handed and friendly.

"DomSubFriends sponsored a speed dating event at Paddles."

"Speed dating for dominants and submissives?" he laughed, skimming his open palm against the slick scalp where hair once grew. "What a crock of shit." He stopped himself to change course. "O.K., maybe I'm not being fair here. Did you enjoy it? More important, did you find anyone to *your* liking?"

"I liked a lot of the subs there. But before they announced who was matched for playtime, I left to feed my cats. I knew what each of these guys was into and thought I couldn't meet their expectations."

"I don't come with any set, specific needs and don't make comparisons between mistresses. You could try a few different things out on me to see what pleases you. I'd be like a male toy."

Just what I needed—a submissive Ken doll. "I hate to be in question-asking speed dating mode, but what is it that you like?"

"I am not here to *like*, I'd be in your life to *serve*. And I'd make no demands. I'd be called upon when needed and available, dismissed when your uses for me have been satisfied. That's whether I liked it or not—as long as my hard limits are respected."

"O.K., what are your hard limits?"

"Just excessive CBT and beatings. I'm not into scat but I'm willing, and have found it quite arousing, to be used for my mistress's golden toilet rituals. But only if she finds this demeaning use of me is her fetishistic preference." He smiled with this last bit of information, displaying teeth too perfect to be his own, and ordered another Pinot Noir.

"That's it?"

"Oh, yeah. I don't do forced bi. I'm not a bi-curious guy. But I'm not uncomfortable alongside bisexual guys. I'm O.K. with other slaves and serving my mistress in their presence. There's no problem being up close and personal with another naked man, when it comes to your pleasure. I just won't be made a cuckold."

"You mean you're looking for monogamy in a slave setting?"

"There could be a room full of naked men—as long as they're all submissive guys I'd be comfortable. I'm just not going to act submissive around you or anyone else if there's a dominant man present. In a group setting, I'd serve and perform around other female dommes and if you are bisexual, I'd act alongside female slaves."

"Not an issue. I'm not bi-curious either." It sounded as if Mister Slave was not a threesome or orgy novice. "Tell me about your last mistress. Was it a good thing?" I was reluctant to sound like those single men who had begun our first date as an interview, querying me about prior relationships.

"My last lady believed the female orgasm elevates and exalts the female, while the male orgasm diminishes him. I abided by her wishes, without question, when she prohibited me from reaching orgasm. She used me in various ways and unlike most mistresses, once we even had intercourse. Just for variety, my mistress would sometimes perform oral sex on me; but if I came close to orgasm, she showed no leniency. Ejaculation into her mouth would be *verboten*."

"Oh, we're on the same page there. Did you two ever go out to dinner or to a party, maybe see a movie together?"

"She didn't complicate matters by doing all that vanilla bullshit. My lady liked to drink so we'd sometimes meet at a bar. Our time together was mainly filled with sex or service. She'd have me make or freshen her drinks. Hours would go by where she'd just tease me, then order me to come be her footstool."

I'd learned at TES-Fest how submissive men made themselves into human furniture for dominant women to sit on, or put their feet upon. "Did she objectify you?"

"Yes and no. My mistress enjoyed tying me to a chair or bed post and stimulating me to my orgasm's edge before abruptly stopping all action. She would do this orgasmic restraint over and over with zero guilt about keeping me in a state of frustration. My torment was her joy." His expression and general demeanor was as if he were speaking of a fond memory.

"You're saying she was sadistic?"

"No, she was just practicing her philosophy: If you control the man's orgasm, you control *him*."

I had heard of, but never fully understood, both the tease and deny fetish and orgasm control. "Why all this denying orgasm? What's the purpose of this—from her point of view?"

"She thought it created a much more attentive slave, and one more eager to be of service."

"Obviously, you agree. Are you looking for the same kind of scene?"

"Not identical. You see, everything I did was strictly for *her* pleasure. That wasn't just how it was—that was how I wanted it to be. I thrived being in such a scenario and got tremendous satisfaction from it." He opened his hands, which had been resting on the bar top, with palms up, as if he had nothing to hide, and wore a beatific smile—one accented by a passionate gleam in his eyes. I'd seen that same look on religious fanatics, conspiracy theorists and political radicals.

But I was attracted to this guy and imagined I'd have to get a BDSM wardrobe to impress him. "Like seeing dommes dressed in dungeon wear?"

"Only if it pleases you. I wouldn't pressure my domme to wear any suffocating leather or latex just because it stimulated me. You do as you wish. And after working a full day, doing the domme thing could be seen as just another job. My mistress should relax; her slave should be the one doing the work, satisfing her needs and desires. Wouldn't you like coming home to change, relaxing, having a bubble bath—perhaps asking me to scrub your back or give you a rubdown?" I imagined he must exercise the persuasive arts for his entertainment industry job, as he was really good at selling me on this.

He just might be someone who was easy to be with. "When you're with a mistress, are you always playing your roles, or can you just hang out?"

"We're always in our dominant and submissive roles, but we're not always in a scene. One of my mistresses liked to greet me at her door wearing a fur coat with nothing underneath. She'd remain near-naked or wear something like a thong, just chillin' while spending our time together. The lady would watch TV, surf the internet, speak or text on the phone, blow-dry her hair—this kind of thing, as if I weren't even there. We'd be together that way for hours, before she'd even order me to touch her. I could never even think of initiating any action, not without her prior approval. Sometimes she'd look over at the boner I'd be sporting and just laugh. It was thrilling for her to be near-naked with an aroused man, knowing I would never be assertive or sexual towards her, not unless she asked me to do so."

"Sure, this would give any woman a feeling of control. I had tea served by some sissy maids. Ever been cross-dressed?"

"I have been, though I'm hardly a sissy slave. Still, I found this a..." He searched for the right words, "a fairly intense experience. One mistress had a big bag of lingerie and made me put a few items on. At first I was incensed—it was something I'd never do and in total opposition to my masculinity. I was just burning up inside, furious at the predicament and at how silly I looked. Maybe that's why she loved dressing me up like that. It's as if she took sadistic pleasure in my degradation, embarrassment and emasculation." He smiled to himself as he remembered these events. "But was it arousing? You bet."

"How many mistresses have you had?"

"Only three, but they were all long term." He propped his elbow on the bar and leaned his face onto an open hand, relaxed in his remembrance. "One mistress would request me to wear sheer white see-thru panties when I met her for a drink after work. I complied, of course. Wearing those panties wasn't the erotic part; it was in satisfying her wishes—even if it meant some humiliation was in order." His panty reverie ended, he looked up at me abruptly. "Why are you so interested in this?"

"Who says I am?"

"You may or may not be into this, as you wish. Cross-dressing is not in my fantasies. But when it comes to satisfying my domme, I am all there for her to control. So if you cared to wrap my manhood in frilly girly wear, that demeaning act would be your pleasure." He hung his head. "It is for me to *endure*." A little dramatic shudder was added for emphasis.

"When being with a mistress, what specific acts did you favor performing, in this power exchange context?" I hoped I was speaking his language, learning to communicate with him.

"Oh, let me see. I am very happy to worship my mistress's butt. At any time it pleased her, she could present her queenly ass to me, her slave, and fully expect it to be serviced and adored. My mistress used to immediately roll over and expect me to lick her hindquarters as she sipped her drink." He smiled while recalling this. "The intimacy of performing anilingus and joy I gave to my mistress, plus my total subjugation—it all came together in such an intoxicating way."

It certainly did sound intoxicating. He'd mentioned drinking quite a bit, when speaking of his former mistresses, and I wondered if a few of these ladies might be alcoholics. Mister Slave and I had finished our third drinks at the Pars bar when the bartender asked if we wanted another round.

"No, just the check." The evening was over and Mister Slave paid the bar tab as a gentleman would. "I realize this hasn't been like your typical first date, where people talk about their education, jobs, and apartments," he commented.

"But I should get to know you as you really are."

"All that set information about your career, neighborhood, family and siblings actually means very little. What I disclosed tonight is what ultimately matters. I hope it gives you an idea of who I am, when it comes to serving my mistress." Mister Slave hopped off his bar stool to stand before me. Ten to fifteen years younger than I, appealing and well-built, he was quite the specimen. We walked out on the sidewalk. "I live right around here and would love you to come visit my kitties," I suggested lamely.

Was there a smile or smirk on his face? "Easily done. I'm a major cat guy myself."

As he walked me back to my place, we picked another day to meet. When I later searched his profile on LinkedIn, he checked out as legit. His entertainment industry position was far different than the work I performed, and so much more impressive there was really no comparison. Mister Slave was who he said he was. But who was he really?

One, obviously, who could lay on the charm. He soon called to set up another meeting. "If you confessed you'd been a porn star, I'd have no less respect for you," he confided. "Knowing that would probably cause me to appreciate you even more." I was intrigued by this open-minded man who was conventionally successful in his professional life yet looking for something off-beat in his private life.

He suggested we get together for a drink (not dinner); but I failed to see this as a red flag because I was so fascinated by him. While being with him on the night we met, he never made a move to wrap an arm around my waist, slip me a kiss or hold hands on the street the way an unsophisticated vanilla fellow would. I imagined this Mister Slave to be very much in demand, one who has seen lots of action, and not needy enough for public display of affection. But as I later learned, this absence of public touching isn't just a signifier of good manners, it's a distinct hallmark of most submissive men.

Neither do they push towards intimacy in the way of a vanilla man,

I noticed as we viewed the colorfully lit Empire State Building from my apartment's living room. We'd gone out to have a few drinks, shared two small plates, make a little small talk. But now we were alone, and what happened next was up to me. As we stood before my large living room windows, I wondered whether he was an exhibitionist. "Do you like being naked when a woman is clothed?"

"Absolutely. Forced to be collared, leashed and naked at my lady's feet—oh, it's the best. All to please her and do what she asks."

"What's it like for you emotionally?"

"It's a feeling that..." Mister Slave lowered his head to mutter, "This is where I belong."

I appraised this fellow who had achieved success in a very competitive career and was at a level that most others (myself, in particular) could never reach. Yet he only felt whole at his mistress's feet. Mister Slave continued to describe more of what mattered to him. "I love pleasuring my mistress orally not because I want to or she asked me nicely. It's like I *have* to, or else. It's when she says, how she says and as long as she says. I do it on command and stop only on her orders."

"How is this better than going down on a vanilla woman?"

"I like indulging my mistress, seeing she's free to enjoy her pleasure 100 percent. She should not—not for even a second—compromise her desires by concerning herself with my needs. I like having my lady totally absorbed in her selfish indulgences, as though she were masturbating alone. This is such a thrilling thing." His voice took on an emotional timbre. "It's just so pure in its power exchange context!"

Either his enthusiasm was contagious or I was ready for something totally different.

Though we'd each had only two drinks, it didn't take much for me to wrap my arms around his neck and draw him close. Mister Slave was responsive but passive, letting me initiate all the moves. Kissing with other men usually led to their pouncing hands on my breasts, then doing the desperation dive up my skirt into the panties. Because Mister Slave didn't push, his passivity ignited something in me.

The scene soon moved into my bedroom. I was used to the typical male demeanor in the boudoir—one of urgency, not deference. If I'd been kissing a vanilla guy while lying on my queen-sized, Southern-style canopy bed, he would have also been trying to get my hose off or undoing my brassiere hooks—all action moving like the Metroliner hurtling towards final destination Fuckville. But there was none of that with Mister Slave. "Would you like me to pleasure you?" he murmured in the respectful but casual way a waiter asks if you're ready to order.

"Oh, O.K. Sure," I replied, not knowing what exactly was on the menu. But I wanted to give this thoroughbred his head, let him run wild, see where he would go. It didn't sink in how I was with a service animal, one who did his duty and only what he was told. I'd long heard vanilla men's comments about past wives or girlfriends who gave detailed, explicit instructions on how to sexually please them—they were referred to as "drill sergeants." But with submissive men, the woman as drill sergeant isn't an annoyance, it's their fantasy! Subs must feel they've been *made* to sexually perform. It would have thrilled Mister Slave to hear me assertively say what I wanted and where, for how long and at what tempo. It would have excited him even more if I dictated he *had* to go down on me *now,* or suffer the consequences.

But Mister Slave sensed this was to be my first sexual experience with a submissive man, wanted to make it a positive one, and forgave my lack of command or authority. He began by giving my inner thighs a few teasing kisses and little licks. As he got closer to my white cotton panties I began to squirm, suddenly wanting more. He continued, never touching intimate territory, until I felt my crotch turn to pudding. "Take them off," I instructed, now consumed by an undeniable sex drive.

"As you wish." His tone was low and hypnotic, a masseur asking whether you prefer Swedish or shiatsu. He lowered them not in a flash, as vanilla men take off panties, but slowly, almost dutifully. I wondered if he was being dramatic, teasing me, or not all that interested.

"Just do it!" Now that I'd given him his orders he was hardly hesitant, diving into my vagina and kissing me deeply there, just the way we'd sucked face a little earlier. The guy really loved his tuna tartare and his face was so smooth, he must have shaved right before we met.

I was relieved my bedroom chandelier had a dimmer switch turned to low light—maybe he wouldn't notice the few gray hairs that sprang from my patch. I imagined he'd never seen a single gray hair down there before. The dude probably couldn't remember snacking on a thatch—girls hadn't grown their pubic hair for the past fifteen years! As I spread my thighs even farther and began lifting my loins, he switched into muff-diving high gear, latching onto my clit like a vibrator made human. Then it was one orgasm after the other with this guy, and he didn't let up until I requested him to do so.

After such prolonged cunnilingus, I had to stretch my legs and one foot found itself against his pectoral muscles. "Would it please you for me to worship your feet?" Not one to initiate action, Mister Slave wanted my permission before performing anything he wasn't instructed to do. He knew I was a fetish novice.

"Sure. Do it." I wondered why Kenny hadn't shown me foot play. But what I did with Kenny wasn't sex—it was sensation and with the exception of my massage, all sadistic acts I performed on him. Mister Slave began by stroking a calf, then massaging my foot before placing each toe in his mouth and sucking lightly. He'd lick between each toe then put a few into his mouth at once. These actions didn't seem choreographed or practiced, but coming from a genuine passion for women's feet. I wondered why no man had ever done this to me before and was surprised by how well I responded to this guy—on his knees, in my bed, with my foot in his mouth.

As he sucked my toes, my other foot halfheartedly toyed with his erection. Though his penis was hard, he didn't press it to me or mention his needs. It was for me to decide whether or not I deigned to touch him or left it alone, even as it throbbed for release. But I didn't want to please a cock that night, it was my night to be satisfied and selfish. These instincts proved correct—I later learned dommes seldom, if ever, perform fellatio on their subs (and certainly not to orgasm) unless it is to tease and withdraw. Dommes don't please, they torment.

I watched him dress. Hardly a gym rat, he was stocky, with muscles where they were naturally expected. His body was unlike Manhattan's typical wiry male, whose pumped-up pecs and biceps oddly pop out of frog-like sinewy frames. I considered how his clean shaved scalp had become the studly slave's favored style and liked the way he comported himself, with a distinct air of masculinity. If I'd once held any stereotype or notion a submissive man would be weak, sniveling or groveling, such an assumption was now dispelled. I was wildly attracted to this Mister Slave—but realized if we were to dance, I had to lead.

When we first entered my apartment, I'd warned him the kitchen was off-limits as I had a sick cat in there. Now peeking in at Orchid's crippled body, lying on her wee-wee pad and double foam mat, he asked, "What's wrong with your cat?"

"She was first diagnosed with arthritis but then she had a stroke."

"How long has she been like that?" He was now fully clothed.

"Seven months. She can move all her limbs, she just can't stand. The stroke left her blind but she's totally aware of everything and still affectionate."

"What does the vet say?"

"He says Orchid is a fighter but if she develops any other serious conditions I should put her down."

"I've kept a few cats. I'd rethink it, if I were you. It could be crueler keeping her alive this way."

"But she eats with such gusto, it seems she wants to live. And if Orchid hasn't given up, I'm not giving up on her."

Mister Slave shook his head. "I disagree. You should see another vet, get some different advice," he suggested in a more critical tone.

"I appreciate your concern, I really do. It's true, she's not going to get any better. But her condition has stabilized."

He shrugged a bit. "Animal abuse takes many forms," he offered in parting.

I held Orchid in my lap for her bedtime feeding. The care I gave her formed such an intimate bond between us. As I scooped up chunks of moist cat food, I realized I'd seen the last of this guy. Not only was I way too old for him, he had been pointedly critical of me and of my judgment. Although a sexually submissive man like Mister Slave may make me wildly responsive, a *completely* submissive man was what I sought.

I remembered what my long-married friend, Carol, advised on selecting the right husband: "Never be with a man who questions your actions. You've got to find a guy who thinks the sun shines up your ass." Carol may not put her feet in her husband's mouth, but he totally accepted her dominance and was ever willing to please. In the vanilla world, this is always a happy marriage; but in BDSM, it is known as a FLR or Female Led Relationship.

Men who engage in submissive sex acts aren't necessarily geared towards being in a FLR. With Mister Slave, I should have heeded the signals. There was no mention of typical couple activities—he'd even called going out to dinner *vanilla bullshit*. Any indication of actually catering to a woman outside of the boudoir was nowhere to be found.

I noticed my panties on the floor, where they landed, and thought about the sex we'd had—sex I'd wanted, enjoyed and now even craved. I help up my panties for a more critical look. They were hipsters, or what used to be called *inbetweenies*. Cut somewhere between bikinis and waist high panties, they sat on the hipbone but weren't as skimpy as a thong. I knew I'd never see this guy again, but hoped he didn't think I wore granny pants.

FIVE

Testosterone Lost

I FIRST STRUCK UP A CONVERSATION WITH CHUCK*, a divorced sales executive in his early sixties, while taking a group class at my local Apple store. After comparing applications, he'd asked if I knew of an affordable, reliable cleaning lady. I recommended he call mine, who could use the work. My phone number now obtained, we kept in touch. The housekeeper soon had a new client and an appreciative Chuck suggested we do dinner as his way of saying thanks.

Safe enough. He asked me to select somewhere near to me so I picked Pars, the Persian place where I'd had wine with Mister Slave. I'd long realized how guys who insist on dining close to where you live are mainly interested in coming up later. Chuck and I were seated across from one another on the pillow topped banquette. "I'm glad you're an adventurous eater," I told him. "A lot of people won't do Middle Eastern."

"Yeah, I like international food. Let's see if they have my favorite soup here." He scanned the menu and looked up after our waitress approached. "Do you have gestapo?"

"Do we have *what*?"

"*Gestapo*," he again said, very clearly. "It's a cold, spicy tomato soup."

Right, it's the cucumbers that take you away to the camps. "He means *gazpacho*, a Spanish soup," I told our confused waitress.

Negative on the cold soups, they had only *borani* (sautéed spinach and yogurt) or blends of eggplant and chickpeas. Chuck, who settled on lamb kebab, seemed to have attention-deficit disorder as his conversation jumped from one mind-numbingly boring subject to another, which included his older son's baby, past camping vacations with his former family, his kids' choices of college, and the daughter's wedding. He also repeated a story he'd told on first meeting. This man was as repetitious as the CNN network news. He was so totally self-absorbed and offered such little conversational interaction, Chuck was the kind of date I had to be drunk to be with. I'd been with too many of those, as my liver would attest if given a voice.

Most older single guys first ask a multitude of questions. (They need to figure out what's wrong with their date so they can more quickly move on to the next woman.) Thankfully, Chuck wasn't an interrogator. During our first dinner, he complained his wife had tricked him into marriage. "Was she pregnant?" I asked. He indicated she wasn't.

When I saw him again two weeks later, he gloated about the wealthy man his daughter had wed. I inquired how long they had dated before marrying, as if I cared. "Just a year," he replied.

Time to go fishing. "How about you and your ex-wife? How long did you date before marrying?"

"Five years," Chuck answered. His only wife and the mother of his children was the woman he had, just two weeks earlier, bitterly accused of tricking him into marriage. After a five year courtship?

I didn't want to encourage him—but when he asked for a recommendation for a trendy restaurant, then suggested he take me there, I didn't say no. I wasn't interested in him, just the new restaurant. And I was fascinated by his fractured front. When Chuck wasn't being the victim, he was acting the saint. "I'm buying my ticket to heaven," he'd say about a dead friend's child he'd "put through college," as though he had money to spare. But on our second date, he told me about this same kid, and how he'd found the time to help him fill out college applications.

"Did you pay for his schooling?"

"No, are you kidding?"

There were tons of inconsistencies like that. He'd laid on the I'm-a-great-guy goo, but not too thick to see through. Predictably, after our ill-advised second dinner, he'd started in. From "thank you for the cleaning lady," it quickly turned into "am I ever going to get a blow job from you?" These words were actually delivered in a distinctively plaintive voice, as if I were depriving him of some elemental human right.

"Look, Chuck, I don't do that sort of thing and you can't expect it from me. We don't have a relationship and certainly not an intimate one. I shouldn't have even agreed to go out with you again because I've recently changed my sexuality."

"What? You became a lesbian? O.K., all right, threesomes are good. You don't hate men, do you?"

"No, not a lesbian. I've become a domme."

"What's that?"

"I'm into dominating men and I only will be with submissive fellows. You see, I have sworn off regular guys like you forever."

"But why?"

"Because they're unreasonable, unruly, too aggressive and just not a turn on. I'm into subs only."

"You have nothing to worry about from me. I'm soft," Chuck confided in a suspiciously brittle voice. "Please, you know what to do. Let's go back to your place and see if you can make it hard for me."

"But it's strictly submissive males for me—and that's not you!"

"I just want to see you masturbate. Besides, I'm so little, most women can't even feel me in there. Whatever you wanna do, doll, I'm yours. You wanna tie me up? *Sawright.* I can get kinky. You wanna piss on me? I've never done it before but it's O.K."

Sex was the one topic where he displayed no attention-deficit disorder—he stuck to the subject. I intended to seem considerate. "Hey, Chuck, I'm not going to make you into something you're not."

"But I'm totally harmless!"

I unlocked my front door and entered my apartment alone. I could always identify the guy who'd has lost a significant amount of testosterone. Their body fat has centered around the vital organs resulting in protruding stomachs, small round shoulders, no tushes and man-boobs. Yet men who are fat all over can usually maintain the old hydraulic function.

I had meant what I told Chuck about only dating subs, and was looking forward to my first date with Stanley* later in the week. I'd met him online; it was a site for men seeking a Female Led Relationship. Stanley lived in the New Jersey suburbs, had suggested we first meet for dinner (not coffee) and seemed genuinely submissive.

"I will treat you like a queen!" he declared when we spoke on the telephone. Stanley sought fulfillment in being submissive to a dominant woman, one whose "word was law" and "wishes were my command." He genuinely seemed both humble and interested in me. Asking the names of my three cats and suggesting I select the restaurant where we'd meet were more points for Stanley. "I am very real but not perfect and am looking to serve," he asserted. He seemed almost obsequious, a most positive trait for a submissive male.

He'd mentioned Italian was his favorite cuisine, so I selected a reasonably priced spot in Chelsea with soft seats. On first presenting himself, I observed a man of about my own age, who wouldn't look bad if he lost some weight, along with the gold chains. After discussing our spare time activities (bridge for me, gambling for him) Stanley turned the topic to sex. He spoke in a hard-charging bombastic manner, and his dinner date patter was probing, as if he were a district attorney at trial.

"So," he inquired. "After you orgasm, do you like having several more or do you pause because you're too sensitive?"

"Oh, I like to leave the table when I'm ahead to cash in my chips."

"Good! See, some mistresses like to be eaten for hours until my jaw gets numb." He leaned towards me, his girth pressing against the table. "And are you a squirter?"

"No, I have several more decades ahead before I become incontinent."

"I mean, do you have an active G-spot?" Stanley crooked his index finger towards himself and wiggled it in a come-hither motion meant to signify stroking.

"No. I don't need to place wee-wee pads on my bedding." The middle aged couple seated at the next table were now so avidly overhearing our conversation they'd stopped speaking themselves.

"Do you know how to stimulate a man's prostate gland?"

"Now why would I want to go and do a thing like that?" A little batting of my eyes went along with the demure Southern lady sidestep.

His interrogation—both in manner and subject matter—made me so nervous I began to fiddle with the ends of my shoulder-length hair. "Don't do that! It's an awful, annoying habit and my ex-wife used to do it!" he ordered. I thought his ex-wife didn't just deserve alimony, but a combat medal. "You know, I can take a lot of pain," he crowed. The man seated next to Stanley, who had been listening to us talk, now turned his head in our direction to better hear more. "I can take a strap-on, too, and a big one. Handling nine inches long by four inches around is no problem." With this, our diner-next-door's jaw dropped in disbelief.

Stanley had insisted the waiter pour me small tastings of three different wines before I ordered merely one glass. "See, I take good care of my mistress. I look out for you, don't I?" I glanced at my watch and wondered how much more of him I could take.

"I get the HIV blood test every six months," he confided. "How about you?"

"I got tested when I had major surgery five years ago. Since then, I haven't asked for it."

"Why not?" he barked.

"I don't see all that much action."

"Do you have herpes?"

"No."

"Good. Because ninety percent of the pro-dommes do. So, do you like to fuck?"

"Only if a man can maintain his erection. Once the signs of impotence set in—no, I don't go there if it's going to be uncomfortable." Most guys never realize how a bendy dick, trying fitfully and clumsily to penetrate, can hurt delicate soft tissue (although a stiff member feels pretty damn good).

"Well then, you're talking about only fucking guys in their thirties and early forties," he huffed. I thought he had potency problems when I'd seen his rounded shoulders and tummy. Then there was all the sex talk. My conclusion? Testosterone had left the building.

"Who are you seeing now?" he asked.

"I have dates planned with two new guys this week."

"So what do you want? Could you be faithful?"

"Well, we cats may be independent and curious, but we still want a home and like to be taken care of."

"So, if you're looking for something permanent, how are you going to get to your goal if you're not being monogamous?"

By avoiding guys like you. Now it was my turn to ask a question. "You've such a powerful and penetrating way of conversing, Stanley. Have you had benefit of therapy?"

"Of course. Years and years of therapy, marriage counseling, encounter groups."

Men over sixty come in two varieties—crazy or crotchety—and Stanley was both. And although he was certifiably kinky, he was not a submissive man, just another control freak. Once home and feeding my cats, I reflected on his initial self-effacing persona, which was in complete opposition to his arrogant behavior.

I checked my phone messages. "Hi there, it's Chuckie. I'm outside your building looking at your window where a cat sits, just waiting for you. Gee, it must be great to have someone who loves you. I was hoping I'd get lucky but guess I'm not a lucky guy. I just want to look at you. I miss those cheeks. And I'm not talking about the cheeks you sit on. Give me a call to say hello. O.K.?"

A genuinely submissive man, not a manipulative, demanding one like Chuck, was desired. I scooped up Orchid and put her in bed next to me, where she usually spent the night. Usually a silent cat, she had earlier growled when I massaged her belly for elimination. I thought she had another bladder infection and planned on taking her to the vet.

The next morning (on a Sunday) Orchid began incessantly meowing, which is termed "vocalizing," while also twitching. I then called my friend, who lived with her husband and three cats, asking for her advice. As most vets are closed on Sundays, she recommended we visit a 24-hour veterinary emergency room. Now on the street with Orchid in her carrier, I hailed a taxi.

We were immediately seen by a vet who examined Orchid, took her history and confirmed she was going downhill. He did the if-this-was-my-cat routine and recommended euthanasia. I watched as he put the IV catheter in place which would deliver the diazepam, propofol and euthasol necessary to put Orchid out of her misery. It was amazing, the vet had noted, how this blind and crippled cat was so fully aware of everything. My tears becoming uncontrollable, I sensed Orchid knew she was dying and believed this was what her plaintive meows begged for. She needed my help out of a life that had suddenly become too miserable to bear.

"You're my angel and we'll always be together," I told her as she was euthanized. To make good on my promise, she was buried at Hartsdale Pet Cemetery, where a pet owner's cremains could be buried along with their animal companions. I'd scouted plots at suburban Hartsdale a few months before, and had bought one on a hill beneath a shade tree. I wanted a grave like my queen-size bed—big enough for me and my three cats—and now I had one.

SIX

Pain Sluts

PERHAPS A SUBMISSIVE GUY WOULD VALUE ME more if he were a decade older, someone around seventy. There was Robert*, an older Orthodox Jew I'd met through Kenny at TES-Fest. He'd been garbed in black with all the Talmudic trimming—wide-brimmed hat and too many layers of clothing. Widower Robert seemed willing to please in many ways. According to Kenny, Robert was a religious Goody Two-shoes who was into being spanked, his only kink. They'd met when frequenting a spanking club. A spanking club? I asked whether there was one in Manhattan.

Actually there were two, explained Kenny—the S.C.O.N.Y. (Spanking Club of New York) and another formed by a former disciple of S.C.O.N.Y. who rebelled, broke away, and formed her own spanking club. I wanted to visit a spanking club with Robert and asked Kenny for his number. Kenny insisted he first call Robert, asking his permission to contact me. (People in the lifestyle are both discreet and protective of each other's privacy.)

Robert called a few weeks later, explaining how he was a very observant Jew. For this reason, he couldn't venture into Manhattan for an early Saturday night rendezvous until November, when daylight-saving time had ceased. (He refused to travel on the Sabbath, which ended at sunset.) Neither could he have any money on him. When I prodded him to explain, he detailed: "Before Shabbat we put things like money and keys to our workplace into our *mooktsah* drawer, where they stay until the end of Shabbat. Then these things are no longer *mooktsah*. The only exceptions to this would be if a life was in danger." I admired his commitment to our mutual faith and promised I'd meet him in November for another kind of discipline.

A few months later, on a dark, moonless Saturday night, I walked to the spanking with Kenny and Laura. The long-wed couple explained some rules. Laura was neither a spanker or spankee, but accompanied Kenny to S.C.O.N.Y, which was open to non-spankers such as herself. It was also one of Kenny's more tame BDSM activities. "Ms. Margaret, who runs the club with her husband, requires no woman call herself mistress," Kenny declared.

"Oh, no goddesses or dommes, no masters or slaves, either," his wife added.

Kenny further explained Ms. Margaret has attendees identify themselves as tops, bottoms or switches. He added that she wants no S&M activities in her spanking club and forbids ropes, chains, studded collars or any kind of gear which references bondage. Good old fashioned over the knee style spanking is encouraged.

On entering the club, Kenny introduced me to Ms. Margaret, a pretty redhead in her fifties, who informed me of more rules. "No pandering or prostitution. No cameras or recording devices. No frontal nudity. No latex, diapers or cross-dressing." She gave me a name tag choice of three different colors, according to what role I wished to play. "Your name?"

"Mistress Pussycat," I answered, forgetting how Kenny had specified no *mistresses* were allowed. Ms. Margaret rolled her eyes as she wrote Pussycat on the red bordered tag for tops. I made a mental note to avoid those with white name tags, the switches, as I was a spanker, not a spankee. The blue border tagged bottoms were more my style. I looked about the room of nearly 60 people and noticed an even ratio of men to women. Longtime attendees Kenny and Laura had mentioned the group was strictly heterosexual.

While waiting for religious Robert to appear, I sipped a Spanish red wine someone had brought and was approached by a few men. (Contribution to a communal food table by every attendee was encouraged; Kenny, Laura and I had each brought something.) Half the men were there looking to be spanked; many of the others (tops) had brought someone with them. A few unescorted male tops made their way over to me, expectant smiles on their faces, only to discover my name tag also identified me as a top. These disappointed gents barely said "hello," when they were there to spank and realized it wouldn't be by me.

I chatted with a college boy from a nearby school; it didn't take much small talk to see he wanted initiation into that fictitious fraternity for subs—I Beta Thigh. I took this cutie into one of the dozen plus black curtained privacy cubicles and went over the safety rules. Uttering the word "yellow" or putting a hand on the ankle meant ease up; saying "red" signaled one must stop immediately.

No time was wasted by the college boy, who dropped his jeans and bent over, his pale bare bottom arched in anticipation. As I flailed him, he squirmed a bit before soon requesting "harder." I was using a black patent leather rhinestone-studded paddle (one more for show than functionality) before I tossed it aside and used my open hand to pinken his buttocks. From taking a TES-Fest spanking workshop, I knew how to find the "sweet spot" that makes a man's tushie tingle. *Cup and lift. Aim for the area low on the buttocks where the cheeks part.* I remembered to alternate buns and not provide a boring, steady rhythm easily anticipated. To say some men enjoy a little over the knee spanking is an understatement akin to saying some fellows enjoy sex. Many guys who are into being spanked can orgasm from it, with no genital stimulation involved. But I wasn't in the black curtained room with college boy for more than a few minutes—I didn't want to miss the arrival of religious Robert.

While I was waiting for Robert, Kenny lent me a few of the several leather and wooden paddles from his duffle bag (which also contained whips and canes). Several fellows there had asked me to spank them—both before and after my session with the college boy—but I gave them all a pass. I told them I was waiting for my friend. When the grizzled and gray Robert finally arrived and came over to hug me, onlookers may have asked themselves *what has he got?* Robert was a pleasure to be with, and spank. Schooled in Europe, he observed how many older guys now into spanking were from another country, one where paddling had been practiced in elementary school. Talking during class, being sarcastic to your teacher, not living up to your intellectual potential, anything could provoke a spanking. For many, being walloped on the buttocks triggered some powerful youthful memories. At a ClubFEM party, I'd met an Englishman who loved to be spanked. He remembered how his nanny had often applied the hairbrush after he'd been naughty. "What do you get out of it now?" I asked Robert, between strokes of Kenny's leather paddle.

"Sexual pleasure," he moaned, his legs twitching as I hit those old buttocks in a certain rhythm, one rapidly gaining speed.

"You can go harder!" he gasped, as the sensation began building. "You can use the wooden paddle!" When bent over, it was amazing how much his buttocks looked like the college boy's, even though Robert had fifty years on him!

After the spanking, we bid our goodbyes to Kenny and Laura; Robert walked me home. Clearly besotted, the religious widower called me several times to suggest dinner dates or other meetings. But Robert lived on Social Security, ate only at kosher restaurants and couldn't afford dental implants.

If Robert wasn't for me, perhaps submissive Benjamin's* situation was better suited to my aspirations. Benjamin had the ideal Manhattan upscale co-op and high-end employment (bona fide Financial Class, at a top-tier Wall Street firm). While first sniffing around each other, speaking on the phone, I could tell he was not impressed by my seedy profession or middle-class address. My perky chat kept him somewhat engaged; but his interest only came alive when I told him I'd taken a workshop in CBT (lifestyle acronym for cock and ball torture).

"You took a course in CBT!" he exclaimed, in an awed tone. He sounded like a foodie who'd just heard his date had trained at Le Cordon Bleu. "Where did you learn?"

"At a TES-Fest workshop."

"And have you ever practiced CBT outside a class?" he queried, as if he were interviewing a recent college grad for a trainee position.

"Of course!" I'd only taken notes during the CBT lecture, observed what our nurse instructor had done to her volunteer demonstrator's penis, then later performed a whirlybird on Kinky Kenny.

Benjamin now expressed how he'd like to know me better. Though he never called me again, he soon sent a text message asking me out. It was the first of two clear warnings I did not heed—he did not telephone me, make personal contact or want to hear my voice. Second, he didn't have me choose the restaurant. Instead, he would text: *Can you meet me at the Bistro Thursday night at seven? Please confirm.* Benjamin was cut and dry, cold and businesslike. He was abrupt when I called him to accept, as if he were in the middle of something. Wall Streeters lay on the charm the way they tip—only as needed but much more to those who are temporarily important.

But he'd made a reservation at an expensive restaurant. Benjamin spent his Benjamins freely and there was never any public risqué talk, always a relief when there are couples seated nearby on both sides. But ours was such an impersonal dinner conversation (travel, restaurants, current events) it could have been between business associates. At least he wasn't grilling me about my age, career, income prospects or lack of marital history, as did the majority of vanilla men I'd dated. I had to be the one to open up first, so I told him why I'd insisted on a place with soft seats.

"I can't sit on wooden or hard molded plastic chairs because I had my tailbone amputated," I confided. "If the sitting surface is too hard, it jams up my lumbar spine." I actually sat on my sacrum, but didn't want to go into that much detail, just provide enough information for future restaurant selections.

"Did you do this for health reasons?" It wasn't such a crazy question with so much radical plastic surgery being performed, and considering the wild body modification practices among the kinkster set.

"I had a major bone spur on the tip of my coccyx which went undiagnosed for years. Every time I sat, I was stabbing myself. The inflammation and pain went up my back and down my legs. I saw about 40 doctors in the States, but first got diagnosed with coccyxdynia when I went to a physician in Paris. A year later I had a coccyxdectomy."

"In France?" He seemed only mildly interested.

"No, from a neurosurgeon at Johns Hopkins. I'm O.K. now. But for several years I was physically impaired and had real difficulty sitting and walking." I'd been that lady you hated getting behind on the subway stairs, the one who took forever to descend because she could barely navigate the steps. I was the woman who spontaneously collapsed in a store. One may have imagined she was on drugs—actually, it was from pain too severe to take one more step. I'd been the chick you noticed on the street being propped up between two friends and stumbling along in the middle as they walked. I wasn't drunk—the inflammation was so out of control I couldn't put one foot in front of the other to support my weight. During taxi rides to and from doctors or hospitals, I usually lay down horizontally in the cab's back seat, viewing only the tops of buildings the cab drove by.

But I didn't elaborate about this to my date. It was as if he'd already zoned out, as do most men who listen to a woman's medical woes. "There was one thing I used to help my pain; do you know what a TENS unit is, Benjamin?"

His eyes, formerly narrowed in boredom, perhaps with borderline contempt, flew wide open. "Of course I do," he barked, now leaning forward towards me, the starched white tablecloth draped about his rotund belly. "It's a Transcutaneous Electric Nerve Stimulator. Do you know how to use one?"

"I'd used a TENS for years, but I don't need it anymore, thank God."

"Do you still have the unit?"

"I do."

At this, he broke into a rare appreciative smile. "I'd really like to see it."

And I'd really like to check out his digs, I thought, after our second date, a rendezvous selected by him and arranged solely by texting. No sex for this guy, I decided after the regulation bread breaking. But maybe I'd have him give me a massage and perhaps some touching was in order. I imagined there was a barrier between us only intimacy—not sex or getting to know each other—could shatter.

Benjamin had selected a three course *prix fixe* restaurant. The appetizer was risotto in a crème sauce, the fish had another crème sauce and the dessert was loaded with more of the same. Riding in his car service back to his place, Benjamin confided he'd dined at some elegant spots with a lesbian couple, who would join him in a threesome after the petit fours. I imagined both babes had a *cum laude* degree in CBT.

I toured his impressive space, the only one on a high floor, a sprawling maze of rooms. Each was decorated in a monotonous masculine manner, the taste of someone who is repelled by color. It wasn't minimalist or chic but big and blah. We walked over to his living room window for an awe inspiring view, one capable of convincing someone how anything was within reach. Though the bathroom is called the tiniest room in the house, his wasn't. Benjamin's can had heated towel racks and tiles, a sauna, a huge glass-surrounded shower plus a jacuzzi big enough for two. Or even two lesbians and a sub.

"I think we'll take a bath together," I told him. Benjamin was too distant to have put a hand on my shoulder or touch me in any way.

"Sounds pleasantly intimate," he declared, as we headed towards the bathroom.

"Having a bath together or even having sex does not make for real intimacy. CBT is taught in workshops; but you can't take a course on how to reveal yourself or be comfortable with another."

"True enough," he admitted. "Tell me what you learned in the CBT class."

"They teach a lot about safety. I never knew a penis could be fractured. I learned how there are two large inflatable structures, the corpora cavernosa. So if a hard on meets up with something hard, if it gets smacked or whacked, all this can be broken. The entire package swells with blood and then you have to explain it at the emergency room."

Benjamin ignored my cautionary words. “I’m not at all interested in having my penis hurt,” he remarked curtly. “Only my balls,” he clarified.

I appraised this man who I thought needed intimacy and, in a sexual sense, knew what he wanted. The guy was loaded and according to him, not seeing any other woman. He’s a rare find, I convinced myself—one who had a sexual quirk but certainly nothing I couldn’t deal with. My response? “Let’s get in the tub!”

After undressing, we lay together in the huge water-filled tub, each on opposite ends so I could touch his genitals with my bare feet. “Tell me more about the class,” he asked, as if he didn’t care to discuss any aspect of life save this. Still, I indulged him.

“They taught us the difference between a sting and a thud sensation,” I remembered, as the jacuzzi bubbles soothed my stressed out shoulders. “And how the upper thighs are way more sensitive to sting than the scrotum.”

“Go on.” He sounded pleasantly engaged.

“They pointed out the underside of the penis is very sensitive to sting.”

“Not interested,” he growled abruptly.

As my foot continued to poke about his sex organs, I noticed he was becoming a bit tumescent just hearing about CBT. I could also feel a fairly small penis atop a large set of testicles. I continued, undeterred. “They said a man can tell whether he prefers either the sting or thud sensation.”

“Not exactly true. I like them both!” he exclaimed, suddenly animated.

I then removed my foot and gave him permission to masturbate. “Why don’t you begin jerking that chicken,” I purred, before adding as an afterthought, “...McNugget.” We had ploddingly spoken of travel and world events through several food courses, yet his penis—no, his package—was the only topic which made him come alive. Maybe this was the only kind of intimacy he’d allow. “I learned thuds are an achier pain, causing the sensation to be dissipated much deeper. But stings are felt in the skin. And there are different toys for stings and thuds.” I stepped out of the bathtub.

His hand was moving faster. "Mistress, may I have an orgasm?"

"You may, but only after I dry off and leave the room," I replied in a gracious manner, as if I were offering canapés to a guest. He's into orgasm control, I realized, while sitting in an adjoining room and wearing a white terry cloth robe which soaked up Benjamin's bath water.

I soon heard a tortured yell and realized the prosperous, porcine Benjamin had attained his release. While taking a taxi home, I reflected on how there's a *quid pro quo*, a give and take, in every relationship. For wealthy Benjamin, "spoil me and I'll torture your testicles" sounded like quite the deal.

At least I have some great food with Benjamin, I told myself as I teetered on too-high heels towards another multicourse fancy feast. He had texted me the proposed time and place at another pricey restaurant, one near where he lived. I surmised he hadn't made plans to visit my apartment because he wasn't really interested in me. But our supping spot was very elegant, the sort of place where men pop the question while popping open the little square ring-bearing box. Keeping this in mind, I put on a vintage Pucci and some of my best jewelry. Although his dinner conversation may be impersonal, even somewhat stilted from lack of real involvement in each other's lives, it was never the kind which makes patrons at adjoining tables blanch, like my dinner with Stanley.

"You know, Benjamin, you should come over to my place sometime. I can make you dinner." I scooped up more truffle sauce.

"Think it'll be better than this meal we're having now?"

"Oh, I doubt it!"

"Then, why bother?"

"Because you can see how I live and meet who I sleep with, my two cats."

"Cats," he sneered. "Dogs, I understand. They're hunters and protectors. But what's the purpose of a cat?"

"Cats are hunters, too. They kill mice. In the Middle Ages, Europe lost more than a third of its population to bubonic plague because people persecuted cats."

"What?" he exclaimed, a fork clanging to his dinner plate. "That's crazy."

"It's true, Benjamin. A woman like me who lived alone and kept cats as pets was likely accused of witchcraft. Being unwed or not having a family made a woman suspect. And if alone and middle aged in the Middles Ages, she was targeted. When a woman was deemed a witch, their cat was called their *familiar*. Cats are also independent—they do not behave in a subservient way to humans, as dogs do. Scores of women, and even their cats, were burned at the stake, sometimes together. Many cats were hunted down and killed, even when not living with a suspected witch. The plague spread throughout Europe because there were no cats left to hunt the rats which carried fleas and bubonic plague. Superstition, suspicion of independent women and animal cruelty all resulted in the Black Death. So you see, cats *do* have a purpose. Now you've said you work with derivatives. Exactly what is *your* purpose, Benjamin?"

"To make the money I must spend on you, Mistress Pussycat," he replied meekly.

"Good boy, now don't forget it." The waiter refilled my wine glass.

After the post-dessert (little sugared jellies and macarons) it was time for the nuts course. "Tell me more about what you learned at the workshop," he prodded, as we sipped after dinner drinks, back at his place. His living room was huge, though not hugely inviting.

"I learned to do the whirlybird," I offered brightly.

"Child's play," he sniffed.

"And they demonstrated parachutes," I continued, undeterred. "See, you have the guy lie down, get a good grip on his sack, and tie it up using a lark's head knot. Then you hang this leather device from it, one having several weights, and if the guy spills anything from his parachute, he gets punished."

"Not interested in games. What else?"

"They taught us a lot about safety. Seems there was a pro-domme in the Midwest who shackled both arms of this guy, put a spreader bar between his legs, then tied his testicles to the ceiling. But then she left the premises and eventually the man fell. After he passed away, she was prosecuted. So they emphasized never tie up a guy's package and use it as a primary hanging point."

"Sounds like good advice," remarked my unfazed date.

"And they showed us a lot of creative toys to use. You don't have to go to a sex shop to get CBT equipment. You can use the pony tail clips, clasps and barrettes girls put in their hair. Our instructor performed CBT with a fish catcher she got at K-Mart. She found some strange stuff, like a brush used to clean hummingbird feeders. And she demonstrated scraping while wearing these long metal fingernails like Freddy Kruger's, bought at a music store, of all places. They were actually banjo picks!"

"What toys do you have?"

"Oh, I have the coolest toy box! It's an authentic vintage smiley bag, bright yellow vinyl and completely round with..."

"What's in it?" he interrupted.

"Some ropes, ties, rubber bands, hair clips, a collar and leash. Plus a butt insert phallic toy."

"Not interested," he interjected.

I had had it with him. "Well, Benjamin, I think it's high time you tell me exactly what you *are* interested in." We sat next to each other on overstuffed armchairs with a side table between us. He leaned into me and whispered, "Do you know about ball busting?"

"Sure. I even saw it being done in the TES-Fest dungeon."

"Think you'd like to give it a try?"

"I have to tell you, I've got such a poor sense of balance," I demurred. "My foot wouldn't make proper contact in the way those athletic girls did it. They taught us not to hit the back of the balls when doing ball busting, as you can cause permanent damage. Because I can't safely aim my foot, we really shouldn't do this." I looked at him with a that-is-that expression hoping he'd move on and change the subject, all the while knowing how a man's sexual obsession habitually consumes him.

"Who says you have to be standing?" he bleated. "Just sit on this chair and use your knee!"

"Look, Benjamin, we took a bath together—for intimacy. Now you seem to be backtracking. How is ball busting going to better a sense of shared intimacy?"

"Because we'll both be unclothed. And all the while you're doing it, I'll be eating your pussy," he muttered, a bit hesitantly.

People who've wisecracked how heterosexual intercourse is the penultimate awkward physical act have probably never witnessed a seated, nude 61-year-old woman flinging her foot and knee at the underbelly of a fat, fifty-something man, one crouching with his head between her open legs.

Men who are bad kissers are no better at cunnilingus. His technique was the sort which begs a reminder: "You don't actually *eat* it." I offered no criticism, as it was the head of someone who has not given much head in his lifetime. He was never even partially erect throughout the act, and his many uttered grunts and groans led me to believe he enjoyed no part of it. But after a few minutes, his sweaty pate emerged from its spot between my knees bearing a soft, genuine smile. "That was the best, wasn't it?" he murmured in a sweet, endearing way, as would a respectful suitor or man in love.

Another guy who just can't eat pussy but tries, and probably impotent to boot, I told myself on the way home. Men who have secondary impotence, those who can masturbate to orgasm but still can't become fully erect, usually seek out much younger women—as if only their vaginas have the pixie dust to make their peckers prosper. Benjamin had a few kinks but basically he didn't ask for much. And if he was with me, he couldn't be just into the young ladies. He didn't embarrass me in public and, compared to many other men, was relatively easy to be with. Could he be the right submissive man for me?

The next week brought another text from Benjamin, suggesting another luxe meal at a designated time. His message ended with these words: *Can you bring your TENS?*

The guy is into only one thing, I groused—having his balls tortured. On the other hand, Benjamin knew what he wanted and appeared to trust me. And how many wealthy, eligible men are there willing to date a middle-class woman over age sixty? Benjamin never asked me if I liked children or why I'd never married, as did so many vanilla men. If he was not on a witch hunt, I would in turn be more accepting of him.

Benjamin just needed some understanding, I convinced myself, as I climbed on my stepladder, retrieving the TENS unit from a high cabinet. As I tested the battery, which proved still good, a sense of gratitude overwhelmed me. During the years 2003 to 2006 I had only hoped one day I could live without pain. My TENS unit had helped. Now I was pain free at last, but using the TENS again to potentially pleasure a submissive. This pain erasure device becoming a pain and pleasure driver was certainly an odd development, but no stranger than many other events in my life, present and past.

I put the nine-volt battery back in its foam cushioned spot, nestled next to the unit and alongside its electrodes and pin connectors. A TENS is used so that continuous mild electrical activity may block pain signals traveling to the brain. In its case, the device is only 8 by 12 inches and fits nicely into a little shopping bag.

Striding into the restaurant to meet Benjamin, I looked like a prosperous lady whose bag declared she'd just bought something chic at Ferragamo, not a domme carrying a medical device to be used as an instrument of torture. The bill was nearly four hundred dollars; but to a man with real assets, this sort of expenditure meant little. Taking his car service up Park Avenue, I leaned my head against his beefy shoulder. "Sleepy?" he responded while straightening his spine.

"Not at all." How long had it been (if ever) since this fellow expressed any tenderness toward a woman? But perhaps this head resting posture wasn't the sort of action a dominant woman would do. I soon donned my new persona.

"Pour me a half glass of cognac," I demanded as we entered his spacious place. "Take your clothes off first. And be quick about it!" The corpulent, nude Benjamin was soon before me, bearing the golden brown liquor in a glass. "Kneel before me," I commanded. "Eyes downward!" Benjamin lumbered down on both beefy knees and stared at my shopping bag on the floor nearby.

"Is the TENS in there?" he asked, hopefully.

"Oh, you're impossible! Of course it's there."

"May I see it?"

He had broken the spell. I was back to being my aiming-to-please helpful self, not the selfish, demanding domme I aspired to become. When he popped open the metal latch and saw the unit, with its adhesive electrodes and jumble of lead wires, Benjamin's face lit up like an underprivileged child surprised with the toy of his dreams.

"Want me to show you how it works?" I suggested.

"Oh, I know how it works, all right."

"Know how you have to put the red wires catty-corner and not next to each other in order to conduct the electricity?"

"Just put it on."

I began by sticking the little pin connectors into the holes of four adhesive-bottomed conductor pads, then placed these on each side of his inner thigh, in the recommended checkerboard red-black position. "What are you doing?" Benjamin demanded, as if something was wrong.

"I'm surrounding the area where you want the stimulation so the electrical play will be felt in the dead center, which would be your jewels."

"But I want the pads placed right on my balls," he asserted.

"I don't think it's safe." Benjamin ripped off the conductor pads I'd placed on his upper thighs and put them directly on each testicle. "Let me see if you've got the right red-black pattern."

"Doesn't matter," he grunted, as he turned the numbered amplitude control up to between seven and eight.

"Maybe we should start at four since you've put it right on your..."

"It's O.K.," he interrupted.

"Beginning to feel anything?"

"Nothing."

"It's gradual," I commented, before seeing his pudgy hand turn the control past nine. "Benjamin, you're going to give yourself heart failure!" I exclaimed, my fingers replacing his, turning the dial to a lower level.

"I'm used to getting it all the way!" His mitt brushed away mine.

"Did you ever have your own TENS?"

"No, a pro-domme would bring it. It was her TENS."

A doctor's prescription was needed to score a TENS unit and Benjamin had no chronic pain. For decades, I had been taken out to dinner either to be publicly seen with the man, to satisfy a courtship ritual, or as a prelude to sex. This was the first time a man had dated me just to get electrical shocks.

Benjamin had turned the control as high as it would go, yet still complained he felt nothing. He then ripped the adhesive electrodes off his testicles so he could more closely examine the potential problem. "I think your wiring is shot. Did you test it first?"

"Only the battery," I admitted.

"How long has it been since you've used it?"

"Five years. I've been out of pain now for five years."

Benjamin didn't care how I had overcome my chronic pain—he was just another sensation seeker. I was well aware how men could use women for sexual pleasure; but this was my initial foray into being used to dish out pain. A few years later, I learned how these electrical impulses can engineer one hell of an orgasm, even if the guy is a total flat tire. Benjamin wasn't my ideal submissive man but a pain slut and one more fish to throw back. And I had let him call the shots, which is not what submissive men want in the first place. I swore that with the next sub I met, I'd take control from the very beginning.

SEVEN

In The Bone Zone

I RESPONDED TO A MESSAGE I'D RECEIVED FROM Billy*; we'd both registered with a kinkster online site. Although Billy had listed his age at 45, perhaps he'd knocked off a few years and was really in his early fifties, which was (I imagined) the age I appeared to be. He'd mentioned travel as an interest (along with collars, body worship and begging) and claimed to have an obedient nature. But I decided to see him because of the questions he asked: *What makes you happy? What are you seeking? What do you like?* I seek and like a man who asks these kinds of questions. A pleaser is what I required.

When we spoke on the phone and arranged to meet, I suggested Chow Bar as a pleasant spot. It had comfy booths in the bar area and served an Alsatian Riesling. The sub, Billy, presented as a tall, cocky 45-year-old with an abundance of muscles. Obsessed with his attractiveness, fitness and health, he worked out with a fervor beyond routine, nearer to compulsion. Billy knew the calorie count and nutritional component of every bite he put in his mouth, one with a lovely set of bleached choppers. He was not only into being perfect, he was all about control and being controlled.

But first came the front. As I bit into my spring rolls, he clued me in to his wealth and success—how he called the shots not only in his business, but in his industry niche. He was divorced, shared custody of his kid with his ex-wife and opined how anyone in Manhattan who sent their child to public school was simply pathetic. "How old are you?" Billy asked. His demeanor was cold and his eyes hard.

"I'm forty-five."

"Then why'd you say you were forty?" His tone was harsh, accusatory.

Here was my moment to change from pleaser to punisher. I reached over the table to pinch and pull his nipple. "Because I'm a bitch! I treat you how you deserve to be treated. And I'm going to make you my butt slut!"

I now sensed Billy's judgmental mind clicking into his submissive head space. "Yes, Mistress," he replied softly in an entirely different, deferential way. I could now let go of his nipple.

"I'm only going to give you the pain and humiliation you need."

His body posture changed along with his vocal timbre—now his shoulders slumped and his head drooped. Initially assured, he was suddenly transformed into someone unsure and even childlike. "What are you going to do to me?" he asked in a vulnerable way, one not the least bit mocking. "Will you allow me to have an orgasm? Please, Mistress. Say you'll permit it!" he whimpered in a desperate tone, as if begging for mercy.

"We'll see about that!" I snapped, as our waiter brought Billy the check.

"Oh, thank you, Mistress Pussycat." Now he was getting the attitude he yearned for.

Billy drove me home in his luxury automobile. But he broke character as soon as he motored up Eighth Avenue, boasting about his big career and big co-op. He asked if I knew what else he had that was so very big.

"Oh, for Christ's sake, don't tell me your big cock," I groaned.

"Your cock, Mistress, not mine."

"Every guy thinks his cock is so tremendous and let me tell you, honey, I work in porn and see cocks every hour of the workday. So what you think is big won't even faze me."

He was suddenly submissive once more. "If your penis fails to impress you, Mistress, you may hit it. Or twist it. Stomp on it, if it pleases you. But please, Mistress, may I show off your big cock? Oh, please Mistress, I'm on my knees! Say you will see it, I'm begging you!"

This captain of industry seemed to be on the verge of sobbing. I had heard of begging as a common fetish but had not yet encountered this sort of intense whining. We were now by the building where I lived and parked curbside. "Well, O.K., then. But make it quick—and you know I'm not going to touch your cock." I wasn't trying to please him, just fascinated to see what he'd do next.

"*Your* cock, Mistress," he blurted as he quickly whipped it out. His penis was fully erect and impressive as promised—thick at the base, narrowing as it rose and bearing an intricate network of veins. The total effect reminded me of those ornate plague pillars I'd seen in Eastern Europe, with all the detailed carvings of tortured souls.

"That's some python you have there," I muttered.

"*Your* python, Mistress," Billy whispered as he stroked himself.

I was mesmerized by the thing. "Just don't get any stud starch on my dress or I'll have to tell the dry cleaner I got sprayed down by a fire extinguisher." His piece was so tragically huge, there was no way any woman who hadn't had multiple births could even entertain the idea of taking it. Just as he was about to spurt, I jumped out of his car, slammed the door and walked away. He'd like this abuse, I imagined, and wondered whether he'd pull out a hankie or possibly ruin his car's upholstered interior.

The next morning, as I dressed for work, a heavily breathing Billy rang me. "Billy, are you touching yourself?" I interrogated him in a strict, accusatory way—as would a mother or Mother Superior.

"Oh no, Mistress," he answered. His voice was one of an obedient teenager.

"Because I have *not* given you permission to do such a thing!"

"Oh, please, Mistress. You left me hanging last night and I'm begging you. *Please* let me have an orgasm!"

"Look, Mister Masturbator of the Universe, I've got to get to my stupid job." *Click!* I hung up on him.

After I arrived at work, I sat down at my computer to research his fetish. As it turned out, such begging and denial, generally called orgasm control, is a widely held kink.

Guys like Billy experience pleasure by giving a mistress power over their ejaculation. They get off on the suspense—will or won't she let him spurt? Ceding power over his boner to another is the bonus. With such a man, forbidding and denying a release is as exciting as achieving it (and maybe more so).

I heard from him again after dinner. The women I played bridge with were gathered around my dining room table. I excused myself to answer the phone in the bedroom, where I could shut the door. Billy was whiny and urgent. "Mistress, when can I see you again? Can I come over to your place? Oh, please, Mistress?"

"No way, asshole. You can't come here, I'm playing bridge. Besides, to arrange a play date first you date, then you play. Next Tuesday, O.K.?"

"O.K.," he murmured.

"I'll make a reservation somewhere. You'll pick me up, we'll dine, then we'll go back to your place. I have to see where you live."

"O.K." He was still breathing heavily.

"Billy, are you touching yourself?" With the door shut, my ladylike guests couldn't hear my end of the conversation or detect my biting, severe manner.

"No!" he denied. "I won't touch your cock without your permission, Mistress!"

I had to end this conversation quickly, so I just hung up on him and returned to the bridge table.

"Who was so important that you leave in the middle of a game?" questioned one of my opponents.

"Senior services." I apologized for the interruption. I'd played bridge with the same sixty-something women for years. I was declaring and took an easy trick but my partner, who was the dummy, didn't place this winning card upright to signify a successful play. The trump card still lay on its side. "Stick it up," I reminded her.

"Such language," she admonished. These were ladies who said "gosh darn" and "pardon my French." My bridge bunch thought I worked as a graphic artist. If they even got an inkling of where I toiled or what I'd been up to after work, I'd never hear the end of it. And neither would any number of New York City bridge players who knew me by sight or only vaguely. The idea of being the topic of gossip filled me with an unease close to revulsion. *Compartmentalize*, I told myself. Accept each of your separate lives—the middle-class, cat-loving spinster and the commanding domme.

It was unlike me to leave a bridge game to take a phone call; but I was both attracted to and repelled by this complicated man. While he loved to be toyed with, I got off on creating different behaviors in him, fascinated by his abrupt character switcheroos. He'd be overconfident one minute and confused little boy lost the next, which only exacerbated my newfound haughty, creative dominance. As a consequence, I responded to him as I had no other submissive man.

I'd seen a review of a new Italian restaurant, one I was curious to try, and made a reservation. On Tuesday, Billy motored by the walkway which connected my building to the street, the timing coordinated by our cell phones. His vehicle loomed ahead as I trotted over on a pair of sensible, medium height heels. I'd taken care to spray my legs with body makeup, covering the broken veins I'd gotten through acupuncture treatments. Just six years before I'd also undergone prolotherapy (delivered through needles), cortisone injections (more needles), a course of oxygen infiltration (six weeks of even bigger needles). Hell, I was the one woman in Manhattan who'd had more needles than pricks! My heels weren't the highest but with what I'd been through, I was grateful to be walking upright. A small purse was in one hand, my vintage smiley bag in the other. A breeze caught the hem of my leopard print silk sundress and carried the scent of my animalistic vintage perfume, a mix of ambergris (created from dried whale vomit) and civet (culled from the anal gland of a jungle cat). I was ready to play.

"Hello, Sweet Meat," I purred as he opened the passenger side door for me.

"Mistress Pussycat!" he gulped, now noticing the bright yellow vinyl bag bearing a grin. "What's in the bag?" His attitude seemed eager and juvenile, but also a bit apprehensive.

"You'll see," I teased, "if you're lucky." He started the engine and pulled out into traffic. I then gave him directions to the dining establishment I'd chosen, in Tribeca.

Everyone should have a secret life, I thought to myself, as I licked the last drop of dessert (a white chocolate mousse paired with candied eggplant) from my lips. I then instructed Billy to ask for the check: "You pay, I say." It would shortly be playtime, or at the very least, show and tell. All through dinner, he'd alternated his persona—sometimes the bad little boy, then the heavy hitting business boss—as if he were a split personality. I wondered what triggered these noticeable changes. Was it something I said or was this all coming from him? I was fulfilled not when a man was in my bed but under my microscope, and didn't like pleasing them as much as observing, evaluating them. There were a great number of submissive men who could serve this purpose, though I'd been relating to men this way for several decades.

Later in the evening, Billy led me into his co-op through the side entrance. Did he think if he avoided the main entrance, I would never figure out where he lived? As if I even cared—he was deluding himself. Dommes can be selfish, egocentric or even egomaniacal, but they aren't stalkers. There are too many fish in the submissive sea. Neither do dommes become too emotionally attached. Blackmail? Yes, this is done by dommes, in some cases—but as a male-instigated fetish.

Getting just a glimpse of the impressive lobby, we were now up in Billy's luxurious lair, which matched his car and attitude—trying hard to be grand. He was proud of his roomy domicile, telling me the name of his decorator, how much the new floors cost, what he paid for the place versus how much he could get for it. He'd also done quite a lot of bragging during dinner. The guy had to be taken down a notch, which was exactly what he was asking for. "Take off your clothes," I ordered.

Billy clicked into his sub space and began to shed his shirt, shuck off the loafers, drop those trousers. "See this roll of fat?" He pointed to a small fold of skin beneath a broad, nearly hairless chest, a negligible flaw in one who could stand shirtless, greeting shoppers inside an Abercrombie & Fitch store. "I'm a few pounds over," he nervously noted, as if seeking my approval. "But I promise you, Mistress, in one week's time, all those extra pounds will be gone. I'm going on a super strict regimen." He pinched his midriff under the perfectly chiseled six pack. "And then I'll be perfect."

If he were a girl, he'd be anorexic. I eyed the gym-trained muscular body standing before me wearing only a pair of briefs. "Lose the tighty whities," I muttered. The python was out now and already engorged, as if it had eaten a mouse.

"You need correction," I sneered. Still dressed, I slithered out of my white cotton Hello Kitty bikini underpants, one with a big cat's face printed on the backside. "You're always yammering about the New York Stock Exchange. Well, welcome to the New York Panty Exchange." I grabbed his briefs from where they were dropped and threw my panties in his direction. "Put these on."

"Yes, Mistress." He donned the girlish panties while I pulled up his jockey shorts. Billy's erect penis peeked out the top of my Hello Kitty panties as he watched me reach for Smiley. "What are you going to do to me?" His voice was as tremulous as a thirteen-year-old's, cracking as it adjusted to a more mature pitch.

I unzipped the big yellow bag to retrieve a small leather paddle. He was lucky I didn't bring a wooden one. "Here's the deal. I spank, you yank. Now bend over." Billy assumed the position, putting both hands on his knees to receive the first few blows. "I'm going to beat all the arrogance and entitlement out of you!" Though he wasn't even being hit hard, his dramatic screams indicated a fantasy realized. "Didn't you hear me? That's *my* cock! And you're going to yank it!" He began to masturbate while I spanked his bottom, still clad in my Hello Kitty panties. "Now tell me how you're going to be my butt slut."

"I'm going to be your butt slut!" he hollered.

"Say it a few more times." Between his many high volume cries, Billy repeated this over and again. I reached inside Smiley for some lube and a purple nitrile exam glove, which looked quite nursey. I'd pinched a box of those purple beauties from Johns Hopkins Hospital when I'd had my tailbone amputated five years before. Billy turned around to look as I put a glove on my right hand and dipped my index finger in a jar of Vaseline.

"Keep yanking *my* cock!" I snarled as I inched a gloved finger into his anus. My other hand reached around his torso and found a nipple to tweak.

"Oh!" he cried dramatically, as my gloved finger crept further inside his canal. "Oh, Mistress!" I began to wiggle my digit inside him. "I feel so *owned*!" He began to beg again. "Please, just tell me that you own me."

I twisted around the finger I had inside him. "You're my bitch, Billy. And I'm going to make you my butt slut."

"I feel like I'm being fucked," he gasped. His hand was now a blur as he masturbated. "Mistress, do I have your permission to orgasm?"

"Not now," I answered coldly, jabbing my index finger up his rectum as I pulled on his nips.

"Oh, please, Mistress, I'll be so good. May I please have your permission to come?"

"It depends. That's *my* cock so I say where you drip that popsicle. Got it?" I spun my index finger in him—it was as high as it was ever going to get—while he uttered some little cries.

"Please, Mistress. Oh, I feel so owned. Tell me where to leave my load."

"*Your* load? That's *my* load you unworthy butt slut. I think you should shoot *my* cock snot over there on your plant. It looks rather undernourished." I suddenly removed my finger, which prompted another scream.

Still wearing the Hello Kitty panties stretched about his thighs, Billy scampered over to a potted plant placed on an end table and spewed on its soil. He looked abashed as he turned around and watched me strip off the purple glove.

I had to keep him in the scene, tough to do after a man ejaculates. "Lookie, cookie, I don't know if you'll ever be worthy of being my butt slut. But I'm going to e-mail you a link to where you can buy a set of anal plugs."

"Plugs? Do I have to have *that*?"

"Billy, you asked to be my butt slut. Right?" I zippered Smiley shut. "Well, you're too tight. You have some training to do. You've got to loosen up. Isn't it your special little wish for me to take you with a strap-on?"

"Yes, Mistress Pussycat." He lowered his eyes and hung his head.

"Well then, work on it." He could hardly have handled rectal penetration by a domme with sharp talons and was lucky I couldn't grow long fingernails. And if he was writhing on just my finger, he couldn't handle a strap-on.

"Don't bother to get dressed or drive me home. Just hand me a twenty for the taxi, that will do." I pulled down his jockey shorts I wore, stepped out of them, picked them up and threw them squarely in his face. Billy reached for his wallet.

I left my Hello Kitty panties there as a sticky souvenir. Billy was good to practice on, but he wasn't what I desired sexually. Though he was certainly a submissive man, he wasn't like Mister Slave, who had this servile, eager to please vibe which just floored me. With Billy, I was just servicing another guy and catering to his kinks, which was most definitely *not* what I sought. But I was willing to gain some experience, add a notch to my strap-on belt.

It would be a long dirt road ahead before I could wield such a thing. Only two months earlier, I'd attended a Strap-On Party at ClubFEM. As I'd left the scene well before any serious play had begun, I'd seen only the demonstration. The party began as any other ClubFEM event—you enter, pay and receive a leash which you may attach to any man's collar sporting a purple ribbon. You snack. Chat. I noticed a new and attractive guy who was opening wine bottles, a fellow in his early fifties who sounded as if he were Eastern European. I imagined his name to be something like Slavko*. But I never got the chance to attach my leash to his collar—Slavko was there with his leather-clad mistress and they were the demonstrators.

Beneath his fashionable all black clothes and skinny pants, Slavko wore a garter belt and panties. I was not surprised—after all, I was at ClubFEM. His mistress informed the roughly five dozen assembled partygoers how anal penetration stimulates the prostate gland, leading to great pleasure (and orgasm) in many men. A regular milking of the prostate was an important safeguard against prostate cancer. But mainly, she advised, some guys like to get poked in the rear because it feels good.

The middle aged domme demonstrator, who was wearing a leather harness around her waist, then placed a sizable dildo into the belt front. She noted her slave was used to something large and could take it—but suggested starting off with different sizes, the smaller ones first. She then opened a kit of anal plugs, a full set which ranged from those the size of a tampon to others the length and breadth of a zucchini. (This kit was roughly the same item I had recommended to Billy.) I knew how female porn stars sometimes used butt plugs to prepare themselves for anal sex scenes, but had never seen such a set until that night.

Slavko's mistress held up one item for the crowd to see. This was an acceptable anal plug kit, she insisted, because each plug was manufactured with a hole in it for the wearer to pass gas (if needed). I hadn't realized how wearing plugs for hours on end, without an air passage, could potentially cause a stomach ache.

She then clued us in about the different straps a domme could don and how dildos were affixed to a middle O-ring. While acknowledging leather is sexy, this mistress recommended a fabric strap made out of a seat belt type material, due to its washability. By the end of the session, she noted, it was bound to get sticky.

I took in all her practical information, imagining perhaps one day I'd have the opportunity to don such a belt. She advised how belt straps could be fashioned in two ways—one riding the hips, the other with a third strap between the legs. Our lecturer informally polled the ClubFEM ladies about which they preferred. "I like the two cloth straps on each side of the hips because they are more adjustable," asserted a Junoesque woman. Another domme desired the third strap nestled in her vagina because it was more stimulating. I remember feeling I was such a neophyte and thinking how this must be changed.

When it was time for Slavko to get poked, his mistress first gave him a little paddling—getting him excited and ready for penetration the way a man gives a woman foreplay before intercourse. She then brought up the subject of lube. Applying some to her strap-on dildo, she solicited comments. The assembled kinksters all had an opinion; they were both picky about and devoted to their brand. As the mistress penetrated her sub, he appeared to enjoy her every thrust. Still, he never attempted to masturbate or ejaculate as this was a demonstration for a group, all for show.

What was it with straight men and rectal penetration, I wondered, as I walked the few blocks home from the Strap-On Party. I recalled Rob*, a heterosexual friend who lived out of town and had slept on my sofa bed for a few nights. A very sexual man of my own age, we had no attraction or erotic engagement, just a long term friendship. One night Rob was out partying until three a.m. He'd suggested I join him but I declined, having been way too tired (and frankly, too old) to keep up with him. No drugs, hard liquor or late nights for me—I'd always had a delicate constitution. Returning from his night of debauchery, Rob knocked on my bedroom door, something he ordinarily would never do. "Sorry to wake you, but where do you keep your dildo?" he politely inquired. After confessing I had no dildo, no vibe, no phallic supplies whatsoever—he was shocked, as if I didn't stock an essential like toothpaste or toilet paper. I insisted my houseguest let me get some sleep, having no patience for his sudden anal appetite. He was high, I imagined, and would be back to his more tolerable old self the next day.

A few hours later, while washing my face, I noticed a strange dirty ring around my tubular-shaped sudsing moisturizer. Fearing the worse, I held it to my nose and was overwhelmed by the rank odor of feces over its camomile bouquet. I angrily accused Rob of using my grooming supplies in a place meant for one way passage. He'd taken my toiletry, he sheepishly admitted—but only because he so badly needed something up his ass! Thoroughly revolted, I threw the bottle away.

Billy, another guy who longed for "something up there," would call me every other day, always early with his morning boner. He'd plead with me to let him touch *my* cock, whimper how he wished for a release, and note how powerfully I controlled that big cock of *mine*. I'd read up on orgasm control and learned Billy's begging was typical behavior for that fetish. But now there was "Please, Mistress, can I be your puppy dog? Would you put me on all fours and walk me on a leash? Please, Mistress. I'd feel so *owned*."

"First you have to send away for a set of plugs like the ones I e-mailed you."

"I did so, Mistress, they'll be here soon. I do everything you tell me to do. And I want to be your butt slut."

"And be my puppy dog, too?"

"On all fours for you, Mistress. Can we get together soon?"

"Call me only after you've started training with your butt plug kit." I hung up on him without a goodbye. A man who acts out as a pet seeks unconditional love, perhaps adoration. He needs rules and boundaries as discipline, not harsh physical punishment. Even more than affection, such a fellow craves a sense of being owned.

Although I'd instructed him not to phone me, I'd receive his call almost every morning. "Will you allow me to have an orgasm? Please, Mistress, say you'll permit it!"

"Not now, Billy. C'mon, I've got to feed my cats and get to work."

After more than a week passed, Billy phoned to confirm he'd received his plugs and how his sphincter was "seriously getting into shape." I remembered this little spot in the West Village I adored. We would meet there where the soft seats and mellow wine would possibly make Billy easier to take. This was scheduled for the following Monday, time enough to prepare for a night of eating and beating.

On Monday I strode into the *boite* wearing a lacy black dress that nicely offset Smiley, which swung by my side. Billy received a hasty kiss on the cheek as I whispered, "What's up, Butt Slut?" My orange frosted lipstick, ever so eighties, was smudged near his mouth. But being with him in public proved trying. We could speak freely, as the place was quiet and no one was seated nearby. But he soon began detailing how much money he had contributed to some cause, and went on to name-drop other *bigs* (his term for wealthy or prominent people) with him at a recent charity dinner.

"Speaking of *big*, how's my cock?" I needed to get him back into sub space.

"Your cock is begging for release. Does my mistress like your big cock?"

"Size doesn't matter to me. I've never been much of a knob snob."

He was clearly dejected. "Why not?"

"Because to me, one impudent sub cock is the same as another. I just wonder whether you'll ever be worthy of being my butt slut."

"I'm only getting used to the first model, Mistress. They're graduated in size, you know, but I'm in active training."

We went back to his place, where Billy showed me his set of butt plugs—which he proudly called top of the line, as if they were expensive golf clubs.

I placed Smiley on a bedroom chair. "Let me see you put one in."

As he reached into his bedside nightstand for some Vaseline, I unzipped the bag. "What are you going to do to me?" he asked in a little boy's voice.

I fished inside the bag to retrieve a leather dog collar I'd bought on eBay. "Kneel before me and accept my collar before you put your toy inside." Now by his bed on bended knees, Billy bowed his head so I could place the collar around his neck. Once buckled, I attached a silver glitter leash to the D-ring and yanked it hard enough for Billy's head to pop up from its low position.

"Good doggie! Now stick that little thing up *my* asshole!" Billy grimaced as he gripped the handle and inched the smallest lubed plug inside. "Atta boy! Now turn around for me and wag your tail!" Still on his knees, he now used his hands, going down on all fours. "Wanna go for a walk? Say *arf*!" He barked a little as I patted his hair. The plug's handle stuck out his anus, angled as a poodle's tail. My tongue made a little clicking sound as I led Billy around his bedroom, second bedroom, den, dining room and living room. Walking him about got old fast, but Billy seemed to be enjoying it.

"Wow, I see my doggie is completely naked—we can't have that," I simpered, as would a most indulgent pet owner. "I think he has to wear a little something on *my* big cock." I retrieved a length of inch-wide lace ribbon from Smiley and held it before him. One of my cat's dressy collars, she'd resisted it so much it had been worn only once for about two minutes. Billy's cock was sticking straight out as I tied the lace ribbon around it. Feminizing a submissive man is one of the most humiliating (and exciting) things a dominant woman can do to him. I remembered how well he'd responded when wearing my Hello Kitty panties.

Carrying Smiley in one hand, with a leash in the other, I led Billy through a dining area into the living room, his kid's room (the other bedroom), past the den, and back into the bedroom. He was crawling on his knees, the lace bow still tied around his erection. For the submissive to enter his mental play space, he must be given one task after the other with little variation in attitude, and there is substantial pressure on the domme to keep the action flowing. The guy can't be brought back to earth—the domme must maintain a certain mood to keep him excited. A sub is then in a state of heightened reality and bliss I call *the bone zone*.

"Some dogs aren't allowed on the bed but *my* doggie is. So hop up on the bed for me." Billy sprang onto the duvet which covered his king-sized bed. "Roll over." He executed one complete turn with only some hesitation, as the butt plug's handle stuck out of him by over an inch. "Now get on your back to play dead with your feet in the air." Billy's knees moved forward to his torso, and he moaned when I gave the bow on his penis a little tug. "Be careful, you dog—these paws have claws." I then lifted my skirt, straddled Billy's broad shoulders, and sat on his face.

Though I wore no panties, I remained fully dressed. "Good doggie! Now eat those Tender Vittles!" He complied with a combination of fear and gusto. Billy would never initiate cunnilingus on his own, but wanted to be forced into it. About as experienced as the average heterosexual vanilla man, he was far from inept yet affected an air of near hysteria.

"*Hmmmpppfff*!" His muff-muddled squeals were at a high, excited pitch, as if he were being smothered. I crouched above him, balancing on both knees—his arms were free to displace me and he could easily breathe. He was hardly in the distress his anguished cries signaled, but the sheer psychodrama of being dominated stimulated him. I could then see how smothering was a major fetish among submissive men.

"Did I say you could bark, you dog?" I yanked on his neck with the leash before releasing him from his position between my open legs. "Look how wet you've made me, you slobbering pup! Now get back on all fours!" Billy again rearranged himself to be on his knees, this time in bed. With the plug in place, his anal cavity was expanded to about the size of a quarter. Smiley, which sat on the nearby night table, gaped open as well. I reached into the yellow vinyl bag for my paddle. I had no idea what dommes say when they're hitting someone. "Cats rule, dogs drool," I sternly intoned with every few strikes to his buttocks, while hoping this didn't sound too lame. Although he was tethered to my leash, he was neither tied nor bound. Instead, he was fully free to jump off his bed, pull out his plug, rub his reddening tushie and call it an evening. But he didn't want that, and neither did his erection. Billy was completely in the bone zone.

"Mistress, may I take off the bow and rub your cock?" He'd had more than a few smacks.

"No!" I exclaimed from my standing position beside his bed. "I forbid it! You may not touch my cock or remove my bow!"

"Oh, please, Mistress, may I please have an orgasm? I'm begging you!"

When a sub begs, his excitement is accelerated by his pleas. "You may not complete in my presence." I unleashed him and removed the leather collar, putting it back in my bag. "But I'll allow you to take out my butt plug and remove my bow after I leave."

"You're mean and cruel," he complained, as I reached into his pants pocket for his wallet and palmed a twenty. He was still on all fours.

"I took money for a taxi because I can't have any unworthy dog driving me home with a plug up his ass and a bow on his boner!" I immediately walked out, then easily found a cab on the street.

Guys like Billy crave unpredictability, I imagined, as I watched the taxi meter click away somewhat too quickly, as if it had been fixed. I asked myself what this guy added to my life. He was amusing enough to experiment with, provoking something which made me feel powerful—but only when we were alone, in a scene. For the greater part of our time together, I was an audience expected to applaud his wealth and success. Every woman acts a bit differently with the various men in her life. She settles on the guy who elicits the version of herself she likes best.

Vanilla Chuck would call me, as would Billy. Both men begged, but in different ways. Chuck had just left me a message: "Hope you're having a good day. Just checking in to give you an account of my exciting day, not that you care. Wonder if you're going to be free so you can boss me around or something. Hey, I still think you're the greatest, so I'm hoping just to get a look at your face. So call me. Please?"

Billy was every bit as needy—but with a more fetishistic hunger. "Please, Mistress, may I touch your cock?" he whined. "Will you please allow me to have an orgasm? I know you don't have any time to stay on the telephone with me but, please, I'm begging you on two bended knees—may I touch your cock to completion after you hang up on me?"

"Have you been training? Are you graduating those plugs?"

"Yes, Mistress."

"Well, don't do the biggest ones. It's not necessary. Go with the next size up because it's been two or three weeks now since you've received your kit and you started with the very smallest one up your unworthy ass."

"O.K."

"*O.K.*? O.K. *what*, Butt Slut?"

"Yes, my sovereign Mistress Pussycat, your butt slut will do anything his goddess says."

"That's better. Try the middle plug but sleep with the smallest inside. Do you like the smallest plug, little doggie? How does it make you feel?"

"It makes me feel owned, Mistress. I like how it makes me feel full. And fully owned."

He was panting as we spoke.

"Tell me how you just love to please me and you'd do anything for your mistress. True or not?"

"Oh, yes, Mistress. Entirely true, I'd do anything for you," he dramatically replied.

"Now why is that, Billy? What is you desire?"

"I want to be your butt slut, Mistress. I need to feel owned," he confessed. On the telephone, Billy always spoke with an urgent submissiveness, one which was diametrically different than the arrogant air he often assumed in person. But Billy only called when he was in his sub space.

Soon he'd be ready for my new purchase—an elastic girdle with a circular space in the middle, which could hold a dildo. The contraption sounded just right for Billy—about as much fun as an aspiring butt slut could have. We arranged to meet and I selected an Austrian restaurant I always enjoyed.

The Riesling was late harvest or *spatlese*, as the Germans call it, not so dry. Although the wine was as I liked it, my date's conversation displeased me. His attitude was aggressive and cocksure. While discussing New York's Rent Stabilization laws, he called anyone who didn't own their own homes "losers," while shaking his head sideways in a condescending *faux* pity. Billy just wasn't in sub space, he was bragging again—first about how much he'd donated to his kid's private school. Then there was the expensive seats he'd scored for some upcoming arts event, and how his donations gave him special seating privileges. As he recounted the names of some leading financiers who also often attended, I finished my second glass of wine and realized I was not yet drunk enough to hear this. I stroked the yellow vinyl smiley, gleaming on the banquette beside me, and visualized the strap-on contained within. With my third glass of wine, Smiley's grin appeared to take on a more demented look.

After dinner and in his car, it was hedge fund this, board of directors that, with some upscale real estate talk thrown in, all the while we whizzed up the West Side Highway. Billy had consumed even more alcohol than I had. Once inside his co-op he easily got into his sub space, seeking opportunity for some play he didn't have to pay for. "How may I obey you, Mistress?"

"First kneel before me." I wrapped my leather dog collar around his neck, then buckled it. "Now kiss my feet."

He didn't hesitate to do so, after which I again attached the little leash to his collar. "You're going to take it tonight, Butt Slut." When I unzipped Smiley to retrieve the strap-on girdle, he stared at it as if transfixed. "Look at this dong. It's exactly like your medium sized plug, which you've already gotten used to. Notice how it's made of pliable silicone and not hard plastic. You can't put anything too stiff or scratchy up there. It could cause micro-abrasions in the lining of your rectum and bad bacteria would get inside, which is how you get peritonitis. This won't tear you up or damage your prostate gland."

He nodded, as if in a trance. "So jump up on the bed for me like a good doggie and get on all fours." I raised my skirt to step into the stretchy girdle.

Billy did as he was instructed. "Spread your legs wider." I reached for my paddle to give his buttocks a few smacks. Billy began to howl.

"Come on, this is just to warm you up." I slathered some lubricant on the dong's entire length then placed its tip against his rectum. As he was still tight, I squirted more lube around his anus. Now being entered, I could tell he hadn't been lying about his gradual use of the graduated plugs.

But I wasn't prepared for the shrieks which emanated from him. As I inched deeper inside him, he grasped the upper part of his mattress with both hands. I stopped to ask, "Billy, am I hurting you?"

"No. It's just...I feel so owned," he sighed.

"You're such a drama queen, acting like the NASDAQ dropped three figures in a day." I began to rock my pelvis with the dong attached halfway up him.

"Oh, oh...you *own* me," he whispered.

"I don't know if you're worthy, Billy, but I own your ass." I reached around his thick torso to give his nipple a little tweak. "I. Own. You."

This elicited a little shudder accompanied by more cries and moans.

Thankfully, he had stopped screaming. More humiliation was in order. "You know, I think you should give your kid's snotty private school ten thousand dollars for every inch of dong I've got up your ass. Agree?" After he nodded his head, I stopped moving the piece in him. "Now beg me to fuck you like the butt slut you are or I'll pull it out and go home."

"No, don't go. Keep it in there. Please, Mistress, I'm begging you."

"You're begging me for *what*?" I gave his right butt cheek a little openhanded smack and yanked on the collar leash. "Tell me, what am I doing?"

"You're fucking me. Please, Mistress, keep fucking me in the ass."

Just minutes before, I'd worried how my sixty-something thighs were not as taut as they used to be, and was concerned about their appearance when wearing the strap-on girdle. But I'd dismissed this insecure concern, believing it was my time to try new things. Having never before thrusted into another, I became aware of how the male must feel powerful and in control of his partner's every sensation. Not only did the thruster take the lead, every stroke delivered potential for pleasure—or sometimes possibly pain. Incredibly, this emotional high was within almost every adult male's reach and I began to comprehend the desperate measures taken by so many, just to gain access to this pleasure/power spot.

But I did not share any of this with Billy. Instead, I threatened: "You better put your head in the pillow and use one hand to beat that meat while I'm pronging you, or else!"

His hand soon became a blur and it wasn't long before he peaked, dramatically screaming "mommy!" a few times as he shot all over his duvet.

Mommy? Was this his own mother for whom he called at the moment of orgasm? Maybe so—he was a sick puppy who'd recently attended someone's memorial service with her. After I pulled out of him and began to dress, I broached the subject.

"So, you want your Mommy when you come?"

"No, Mistress, I only want *you*." He had now turned over on the bed, facing me.

"You're calling *me* Mommy? Do you actually think of me that way?"

"Uh-huh. Sure. Don't you? Aren't you...mommy?"

"Only to my cats," I replied, now feeling humiliated myself. "I can't believe you think of me as *mommy*!"

"Look, I know what I am." Billy quietly declared, as he pulled the bed sheet about his well-developed torso. "But do *you*?"

Of course, after their orgasm, men are no longer in the bone zone and reality rears its ugly head. Stuffing the dong in a plastic bag, I dressed in a flash to beat a hasty retreat. Now hailing a cab with Smiley in hand, I'd even forgotten to take taxi money, I was so horrified. And why wouldn't the guy think of me as mommy? As he was 16 year younger, I must have seemed like the mother of a cougar.

Billy would call me up and ask me out from time to time, but never regularly, and I always declined. His interest was too spotty and erratic. Men are like shits—they have to be regular. But all that went down with Billy increased my sense of competence in dominating men, which I sought after my debacle with the ball busting Benjamin. Billy hardly met my needs—my time with him was too much like unpaid sessions.

During this period vanilla Chuck kept calling, asking whether he could take me to one swell eatery or another. I remembered the men I'd dated over the past three decades: the beautiful porn studs I'd bedded in the eighties; the prosperous yet porcine potential husbands I'd gone out with in the nineties; and now, submissive men.

I'd gone from studs to schlubs to subs.

EIGHT

My Kinky Sock Hop

I'D LONG HEARD VANILLA FELLOWS DISAPPROVE of women who "have an agenda," basically male-speak for making reasonable demands. But men have an agenda, too, with sexual intercourse topping the list along with frequency, length, and creative quality of the act. Mere access to the honey pot was enough to satisfy a man 30 or 40 years ago. Now with the pervasiveness of limits-pushing pornography, even the most average guy demands a nether region shaved bare, an anus willing to be penetrated, and a pliant body ready to assume all sorts of impersonal sex positions (such as the pile driver).

Submissive men aren't like that—the vast majority don't crave fellatio or even want conventional sex. This doesn't mean these subs have no needs or make no demands—their desires are just out of the ordinary. And for many, we're talking way, way out.

Though scores of men described themselves as submissive, I realized they were only *sexually* submissive. Finding the rare gem who said "yes, dear" and "anything to make you happy" would be more likely on JDate. Many of the males who called themselves subs were die-hard control freaks and not so submissive as much as they were masochistic. Where were the manly submissive men?

I had heard femdom stemmed from the medieval Code of Chivalry, an intriguing concept. With this in mind, I attended a meeting of a group called Dominant Women and Alpha-Male Submissives held at my neighborhood's S&M palace, Paddles. Their leader had posted much about femdom's roots in chivalry on the FetLife website. Many dommes look upon medieval knights, who performed feats of bravery as well as routine duties for their fair lady, as precursors to the modern submissive man. More than a few subs idealize this romantic knight in shining armor notion as well.

Over 40 years prior, I'd written a college term paper on chivalry; the road to knighthood had fascinated me even then. I now tried, from what I remembered, to find a connection between chivalry and femdom. Knights came from families of means, yet only the eldest son could inherit land. For this reason, only *he* would wed (at the onset of puberty) the daughter of another well-off family. But pity the several younger sons with no land nor means of support and, consequently, no early marriage prospects. Such landless highborn males were encouraged to become knights.

At the time modern kids graduate from college and go out into the world (age 21) there was a flurry of fasting, praying and several dramatic ceremonies. At their conclusion, a squire (who'd been in training for years) became a knight. The young knight often sported a boner for his liege lord's wife and milady had scores of loyal, flattering younger men willing to please her. True blue knights had some brown noses—praising the powerful lady and denying themselves was their way of getting ahead. Though the lady was wed, this would never stop a knight from declaring his unrequited love. These lords' and ladies' marriages were arranged, never love matches. As a consequence, all the dramatic extramarital wooing gave feudal courts the titillation and gossip they craved. The lady never gave in to her knight's passion but was expected to lead him on in a romantic sense—then into battle, to protect her family's interests. Typically older than the knight, these females were hardly maids, more like medieval MILFs. All the knight got out of it was a certain fame and glory, never the fur box. This practice of what is called "courtly love" was both widespread and socially accepted.

Such extramarital affairs were glorified by troubadour ballads and certain lovers became as infamous as today's reality TV stars. Many lengthy poems detailed the gallant knight's combat skills, good deeds and sacrifices made for his chosen ladylove; he became a medieval celebrity. Especially popular were accounts of a heroic death, the lady's name on the knight's lips, his actual heart extracted from his body and delivered to her in a wooden box. In the Dark Ages, such sordid and sentimental sagas excited their listeners to no end. It was their porn.

Those shining coats of armor shielded legions of blue balls, but sexual restraint was shown only towards ladies of noble birth. If a knight happened upon a wench alone in the field or forest, she was often raped, with no repercussions or reprisals for the knight. And if this peasant girl was from a land with whom the knight's lord or king was at war, she was usually dead meat. Courtesy and reverence for women was class specific; chivalry was not extended to commoners.

Although that's how knights were back then, I had expected to see chivalry in action in the here and now, within this group who met at Paddles, simply because the group's leader had posted several papers about femdom and chivalry online. One of the women expressed an urgent, immediate need to find a new apartment. I suggested the assembled men devote themselves to this fair lady's request and help her get what she needed to survive, calling it "practical chivalry in action." But chivalry was not what the guys were there for. As one sixtyish fellow piped up: "Milady, I need a spanking; but can you only hit my left cheek? The right is torn up already, it's raw." As he pulled down his pants, bent over and got his saggy old ass royally walloped by a thickset woman wielding an equally thick paddle, I realized a lot of the men present were just heterosexual masochists looking to get their needs met.

I watched as the pallor of his left buttock began to take on the same mottled red palette as a bowl of Chef Boyardee Beefaroni and realized I was not inspired by the males within this club. It wasn't that I was unfamiliar with dingy places. The unimpressive job, long days on dreary porn sets, plus reporting on the peep shows, strip clubs, swing parlors and cat houses I'd frequented had allowed my desired Manhattan lifestyle. I was hardly compromised: I naturally gravitated to offbeat people and experiences. And as a provider of stability and financial security, pitsy places and porn was an acceptable substitute for the more traditional loveless marriage.

Most of the men outside our little group were dominant males cruising for a female tushie to whack with rod, whip, palm or paddle. Though their look was Seventies Village People with lots of studs and leather, their initial approach and demeanor was as sunny and unthreatening as a Sunday school teacher. "Hi there, are you a bottom?" they'd inquire in an upbeat, chipper tone, an open smile beneath their mustache or above their Mephistophelian goatee.

"No," I'd reply, "I'm a top." Their smiles would melt and backs turn to walk away. There was no top-to-top or dom-to-domme camaraderie between men and women—these doms were strictly seeking fresh meat to beat.

As I walked about the club, observing the suspension bondage setup and how the leather cuffs attached to the chains, a short, bald, middle aged man scurried over and prostrated himself before me. "Mistress, may I kiss your feet?"

"Not now," I replied curtly. Much later that evening, I'd ask myself why I denied giving him the pleasure of kissing my well-worn comfort shoes, hardly an intimate act. It was many months later that I began to understand how rejection would be far more exciting to him than having his wishes realized.

I gradually learned how to deal with the many men I came in contact with—through group meetings, munches and also online. There was the sub who said he lived for housework. He'd clean, vacuum and scrub the tub. Perhaps this would sound appealing to a lady who didn't have a regular cleaning lady. In the vanilla world, if a guy takes a girl out to dinner three times, he's expecting wild sex. Within femdom, if a fellow thoroughly cleaned a woman's living quarters for four or five hours, the most he could hope for is her permission for him to achieve ejaculation on his own—she would never even think of touching him. If he was lucky, she just might grace him with her presence, or be in the same room when he exploded into a Handi Wipe. While vanilla men get huffy or feel exploited if they don't get sex within a certain time, true submissive men make no erotic demands and are even turned on by their rejection.

And rejection is just what the typical submissive man is used to. My latest contact was a suburbanite whose WASPy looks matched his mild but persistent manner. I kept in touch with Kevin*, a corporate type of about my own age, who spoke in middle management lingo. He didn't want to talk but *dialogue*. He needed to *reach out,* he'd say, *touch base*, or give me a *heads up*. With all the business speak, I was expecting a future performance review. Instead he offered, "I'm onboard meeting you anywhere you like, and wearing a diaper on the inside or outside—your choice." Kevin said he'd drive into Manhattan and while we were out and about, he'd wet his diaper so it would get all soggy and smelly. He assured me this would excite us both.

To register a protest, I reverted to my old Southern lady self. "But I wouldn't want to have you catch a cold in the dead of winter."

"I'll wear my flannel diapers," he replied matter-of-factly, without a trace of irony.

"Well, it's just that...if you wear such a thing when out with me, I'll have to kill you."

"Oh, O.K. then," he grunted.

He's my age, says he's divorced, sounds very submissive, let's make plans. When I suggested we should get together for a drink, he countered how he didn't know many locations and wouldn't be able to find our meeting place, even if I gave him the address. I'd met Kevin at a Manhattan munch—surely he knew how most streets are laid out in a grid. He also claimed an unfamiliarity with the subway system and instead wanted to hook up around the Lincoln Tunnel. I explained there were no places right around the tunnel (unless transvestite hookers were to be entertained in your automobile's back seat) and instructed him to arrive on the train. We exchanged cell phone numbers, then agreed on a time and place somewhere near Penn Station.

He'd noted how he loved seeing the city's impressive seasonal decorations. "The best walk for seeing the Christmas lights is up Fifth Avenue," I suggested. "We'll stop for a drink on 57th Street, after which we'll walk two blocks west to the Time Warner Center." Kevin had never seen these twin towers; I briefly described the architecture with mall and fountains surrounding the lit statue of Columbus outside.

As he was a submissive man, I thought he'd like being told what to do. But a few days later, he called to ask why we were going to a mall. He instead lobbied for somewhere else: he had other plans for our evening together. Kevin was into karaoke, supposedly had a good singing voice and wanted me to accompany him to a bar, waiting for several hours at an amateur night until he got his turn at the mic. Listening to your guy warble Tony Bennett tunes to drunk strangers is something a well taken care of wife does, and only if hubby has earned it. But on a first date? I was seeking a Female Led Relationship where the woman did the controlling, not the guy! Though he claimed to be a sub, Kevin was just not into pleasing me. I canceled our rendezvous and gave him no encouragement for further contact.

Then there are the subs with very specific sexual fetishes who are seeking a woman specifically into the exact thing. "So does it turn you on to watch a guy put on women's clothes, makeup and wear a wig?" asked one man over the phone.

"I get satisfaction seeing a man realize himself. If I like him, and that is what turns him on, I'll get pleasure just by being involved," I babbled to this cross-dressing interrogator.

"Well, you make it sound like some kind of a trade-off!" he pouted in a critical tone. His dissatisfaction was clear. Subs have fantasy expectations of women the way vanilla men do. In the same way guys can dream of preternaturally orgasmic women ("she comes if you just stroke her forearm") or mutual orgasm ("we always come together, we're so much in tune"), many male subs expect women not just to appreciate their sundry fetishes but to be driven by these same obscure desires. ("Do you like to fart in a guy's face while wearing a cheerleader uniform?" "Crave administering chocolate milk enemas while tying up testicles?" "Love squishing big bugs with your stiletto heeled gladiator sandals?")

Who cares, mister—you're lucky if you can get a lady to be in the same room with you!

But something more important than working by day and frolicking with submissive men at night was demanding my attention. Suddenly I couldn't see well out of my left eye. At the hospital retinal clinic, a doctor shined a blinding white light in my eye. (I imagined this could be the sort of thing they'd do at Guantanamo Bay to Islamic terrorists.) It's either a macular pucker or a cortical cataract, declared both the ophthalmologist and the eye surgeon. Unlike the usual nuclear sclerotic cataract which grows on the lens surface over a lengthy period of time, a cortical cataract comes on rapidly and its effects are more severe. Then again, I could have a macular pucker, they opined, a condition which can develop from the vitreous detachment I'd had the year before. They couldn't diagnose me until surgery, so I was scheduled for cataract extraction with implantation of a lens.

During a pre-op visit to the Eye Infirmary, I'd spent several hours waiting for my orbital proportions to be measured. A man in his sixties struck up a conversation with me while we were both in the retinal clinic. "What are *you* in for?"

"Cataract."

"A cataract at your age? You're way too *young*!" His manner was frankly flirty.

"You can get them at any age." The guy was slim and fit, well dressed and attractive. Meeting a normal guy, for a change, seemed appealing. "What brings you to the Eye Infirmary?"

"Macular degeneration," he confided before launching into his tale of woe, which centered more on his failed marriage than failing eyesight. He'd been a very successful designer when he met his wife, who was two decades younger. His friends had warned him to be wary of the age difference, but he'd anticipated no future harm in one with such creamy skin, lithe limbs and general air of innocence. Twenty years later, he was a 63-year-old father of two college-age kids and rapidly going blind. As he'd had no pre-nup and his wife didn't work, he was being sued for alimony with full support. A friend's sofa bed was where he now slept—his wife had been awarded their spacious marital home.

"My eyesight has deteriorated so much I can barely see. So I can't work anymore. But enough about me, let's talk about *you*. You're so *young* to be having cataract surgery!"

"Not really. I'm 61."

"Sixty-one! *Sixty-one*?" he repeated in a tone of dismay. "Well, all I can see is some fuzzy features and the long blonde hair. So I thought you were about my wife's age. My God, I really am going blind," he moaned before abruptly moving to another chair across the room. There he waited his turn for another two hours, safely away from the suddenly undesirable woman his own age.

The evening before my cataract surgery, my girlfriends were coming over for dinner and Denny Vinny* was to entertain us. He was a hunky 38-year-old Italian construction worker who lived in Queens. Outwardly macho, on the surface he seemed too cocky to submit. His self-confidence, strut and accent reminded me of John Travola's character in *Saturday Night Fever*. But burly, jocky, *uber*-masculine types are as likely to be submissive as their beta brethren. It's difficult to spot a submissive man, in the way one can get an indication a man is gay.

My three female invitees had gotten word a naked man would be serving and dancing for us. When it came to putting Denny Vinny through his paces, I would be directing it all. Submissive men may have a willing nature, but his domme must take the lead through tone and attitude. During our first phone call, Denny Vinny confessed how he was into humiliation by a group, women I would hopefully invite over. Hardly coy about what kind of action he was seeking, Denny Vinny was the typical seasoned sub who knows what he wants and readily asks for it. His needs were very specific and we'd had several conversations about what he craved.

"I want you to take off my clothes or make me take off my clothes," he told me in an urgent masculine voice. "Have me bow down to you. Force me to exercise, like they do in the Army. Laugh at me with lots of pointing to my tiny cock, then make me jerk off while you laugh. Fart in my face, please, I'll love it. Slap my face or spit on me. Kick me in the ass. That's all good. And lots of verbal humiliation, O.K.? Also play with or do something to my balls. And maybe you can hog tie me and put an apple in my mouth?"

"You mean like a roasted pig? Sorry, I'm no good with rope. The rest I can try and do." The guy didn't beat around the bush, so neither would I. And he wasn't a pain slut into being hurt. After we'd discussed these matters on several occasions and I'd absorbed all this very personal information, I came to a conclusion—it's party time!

Although Denny Vinny wasn't the sort of submissive man I sought, I wanted to make his fantasies a reality. I approached most subs with the same self-centered attitude I had with vanilla men—how can you meet my needs? But some sweet and sincere chord in Denny Vinny made me want to satisfy *him*. I'd pay for the catered food and provide his audience. But where would I get a group of cruel and demanding femmes?

I contacted a few lifestyle dommes I'd met at parties and workshops, asking them to my affair with Denny Vinny. But these jaded femmes regarded such an evening as mere Mickey Mouse behavior. They needed a one-on-one with a worshipful sub who'd do their cleaning and chores. No domme would attend my *soiree* and see it as a lark. For this reason, I invited some of my best girlfriends, all vanilla and unexposed to femdom. They were already clued in about my new lifestyle; I now warned them they'd be served by a nude submissive man. "Don't come if you're easily shocked," I insisted to Mallory*, a single litigator in her sixties. My octagonal shaped dining room table seated four. Denny Vinny would serve Candy*, Suze*, and Mallory dishes they'd previously selected from a nearby Italian restaurant.

On party night it was all delivered piping hot to my door, and very close to the time my guests arrived. These ladies eyed the decades younger Denny Vinny uneasily, as Candy suggested he uncork the wine she'd brought. "But he has to strip first," I declared. "Take everything off before you serve us our dinner," I casually told him, as if I were asking a sommelier to show me the bottle label.

"Yes, Mistress Pussycat," he responded as he shed his clothes. Mention of this scene name made my friends erupt in laughter, just what

Denny Vinny needed to achieve an erection. For a man who begged to be humiliated about his small cock, he sported a large appendage, one that noticeably stiffened with female laughter.

"Now *present* to receive the house collar," Nude and erect, he dutifully knelt on my oriental rug, lowered his eyes and crossed his wrists behind his back, in keeping with the most commonly used submissive positions. I had known he was an experienced sub from our many talks. Now fastening the leather dog collar I'd used on Billy around Denny Vinny's thick neck, I ordered him to *submit*. Three wide-eyed ladies stopped giggling and sipping, their wine glasses in midair, to witness the naked Denny Vinny sit on his heels and lean forward until his forehead touched the ground. Still prostrate, he simultaneously placed his arms overhead with his palms up and wrists crossed. My guests, all stunned into silence, could think of no other response but polite applause.

After I approached him and threw one leg around his back, he instinctively put his hands down to become a beast of burden and carried me on all fours. As I sat on Denny Vinny, he dutifully trod on his hands and knees around my living room. "What do you think of my horse, Denny Vinny Pretty Guinea?"

"It's better than a Strip-O-Gram boy," offered Suze, a thrice-divorced, hard-nosed realtor in her sixties. The ladies giggled but seemed nonplussed by the pony play, so I dismounted my stud.

"Now let's see you do some push-ups." Forced exercise was one of his fetishes. As he assumed the position and dropped to the floor, I began to count out loud. My guests soon chimed in. Denny Vinny not only wanted to be humiliated, it was part of his larger CFNM kink. CFNM, or Clothed Female Naked Man, is another manifestation of the submissive male objectification fetish. In a wicked role reversal twist, the male becomes a subservient sex object. Men who are into CFNM are always exhibitionistic, but not all have the etched pecs, hard body and sizable penis of Denny Vinny. Guys into CFNM get off on being the only one undressed and in a lesser position of power.

After he'd done enough push-ups, we were ready to move on. "Rise and continue to serve," I instructed in my newly acquired regal tone.

Now having dinner, the girls were mainly interested in chatting among themselves, and paid my nude waiter so little attention their disinterest was almost rude. As he continued to fill wine glasses, they asked him a few questions typical of New Yorkers. "Where do you live? What do you do?" As his job and outer-borough neighborhood failed to impress, they began to give advice about how he could make extra money going into business as a nude butler.

"But he can dance, too!" I enthused before turning to an old tape cassette player hidden behind a sofa. (I'd previously informed Denny Vinny how he'd be made to dance and the song chosen for him was "Cool Jerk.") My boom box blared as the guy shook his buttocks and wiggled his large manhood in undulating circles. The ladies laughed and clapped with each of his moves; they even followed my lead by often pointing at him.

I took one of the vividly colored blowout squeakers I'd bought from a party store and unleashed it towards Denny Vinny's penis. The women squealed as the thing honked and unfurled, its tip touching the sub's genitals. As I passed out more squeakers, each lady took it between her lips and followed my lead. "Joyce is whooping it up tonight because she's going in for cataract surgery tomorrow," noted Candy.

"*Sh-h-h*, not in front of the children." I murmured as Denny Vinny turned his muscle-ripped torso to Suze and her curling, tooting toy. Would his submission be as effective if he knew I was in my sixties? I doubted that.

My guests had reached their limit when I reached into my smiley bag and extracted a long rope with a slipknot in it. "Put this around your little thingy," I said, as I handed the string set to him. It was part of the same raunchy reins I'd used at the ClubFEM Pony Party.

"Yes, Mistress Pussycat," he replied, as in a trance. There were no peals of laughter this time—my girlfriends now realized who Mistress Pussycat was and she was not the well-mannered Southerner they thought they knew.

He put his organ inside the opening—the slipknot was tight enough to secure him that way. The girls were aghast to see me tugging on a rope fastened around his penis, leading this young guy about and pulling on him to follow. But judging from the angle of Denny Vinny's wiener, he loved it. There is some primal pleasure which kicks in when a submissive man is led around this way. Whether it's the friction of the rope on the sulcus (which lies between the penis' glans and shaft) or the animalistic feeling of being dominated, most subs respond well to this love lasso.

As my female guests' mouths were now agape, I soon unleashed my sub and played another old tune. "Know how to do The Bump?" I demonstrated the dance by angling my bottom against Denny Vinny's naked buttocks.

"C'mon, girls, everyone do The Bump!" Soon we were all dancing along with the hard-bodied, ever-erect Denny Vinny. He was having a great time sliding next to one lady or another and bumping her hip or rear. It wasn't sexual or hurtful, it was fun—as most easy to execute retro dances are for seniors—yet I had to caution him. "Don't bump too hard, Denny Vinny, I have some brittle bones." I would not say the word *osteoporosis*.

As the song ended, I realized our nude server deserved a release. Submissive men either ask for permission to orgasm, or it must be ordered by the domme. I actually wanted him out of the house (so I could talk to my friends with no distractions) but thought a wet finale was in order. "My favorite band is The Red Hot Chili Peppers," I told him, "and they sometimes used to perform nude wearing just a sock where there should be a jock." I looked at the pile of clothes Denny Vinny had doffed. "As a tribute to The Chili Peppers, I want one of your socks back on—but put it around your cock and jerk off in it."

"Yes, Mistress Pussycat," he responded with a slight involuntary smile. It was obvious Denny Vinny not only needed an orgasm but appreciated the opportunity to have one that was specifically ordered, and before a live audience.

He wasn't even erect as he reached for his sock and put it on his penis. Suze still squealed, "Oh my God, it's so big!"

But Candy, who had just surreptitiously read a list of Denny Vinny's kinks I'd written down and put on the kitchen counter, was quick to share. "He doesn't want you to admire it," Candy whispered to Suze and Mallory, as they observed the young man pulling his phallus. "He wants to be humiliated!" Candy then pointed to his meat-stuffed, lumpy sock. "It's little!" she shrieked while waving her arm in his direction. "The guy has a tiny cock!"

"It's little!" I chimed in while pointing a finger directly at him.

"It's insufficient!" exclaimed Mallory the attorney, as she wagged a well-manicured forefinger.

"It's minuscule!" Suze followed and in seconds, with four femmes pointing fingers at him while telling him his manhood was under par, Denny Vinny's sock turned from lumpy to statuesque.

"Now beat it! Come in your sock and don't get any gristle gravy on my fine home furnishings!" I thought that imperious tone would turn him on.

"Tiny cock! Tiny cock!" we four finger-pointing ladies chanted as Denny Vinny pulled his peaking penis tucked inside the knit sock. Soon enough, after his hand had become a blur and his face contorted in ecstasy, he ejaculated into the sock.

"Good boy." I smiled at him. "Now put your sock over your foot and wear it on home."

"Oh, no!" groaned my friends, laughing as if this were a silly party prank instead of BDSM. But Denny Vinny put his soggy sock on just as he was told. After we thanked him for serving and bade him goodbye, Mallory turned to me with a steely glint in her eyes. "You said he was going to be subservient, nude and serving but if I'd known it was going to be this rough, I never would have come. I'm an attorney!"

"Hey, I wanted to be among friends tonight and whoop it up before cataract surgery tomorrow morning." I thought of all the fancy Manhattan cat houses I'd visited as a pornographer. Among the young girls lolling about waiting for johns, several had their noses in a law school textbook or were studying for the bar exam. It seemed as if screwing your clients was great preparation for a career where you could do similar work.

"You didn't want Denny Vinny to know about your cataract surgery," Candy noted. "Just how old does he think you are?"

"Oh, I routinely knock off twenty years."

"And these fellows don't question you about it?" asked an incredulous Suze.

"So, you don't feel you owe them the truth. Right?" Mallory interrogated.

"They're in it for the fantasy and reality is the last thing they want," I explained. "You've seen all these divorced men in their fifties dating women twenty years younger. The guys are not getting married, they're just wasting these girls' time. If men consider older women to be desperate, try talking to single women between the ages of 35 and 40 about their childbearing prospects. Manhattan males have long been involved with decades younger females, even before the sexual revolution, just because they can. And what's good for the gander is great for the goose."

"Did you invite us over so you could write about it for your job?" Suze asked pointedly.

"I write as Amanda, a 24-year-old editorial assistant just learning the ropes. The readers never know their Amanda is actually sixty-something, an old lady who's worked in porn for many years past young Amanda's life span. What went down tonight could never be written about for work. No mention of humiliation is allowed in the magazines—we must adhere to strict censorship rules."

"I can't believe how many decades you've had that crazy job," Mallory moaned. Besides the steady paycheck, healthcare and 401K, I could think of one other benefit: when I began to edit a magazine for submissive men, I had found femdom. How many people feel they've discovered their true sexuality through work?

At eleven o'clock, after we'd all said goodnight, I snuggled between my cats and reflected on my party guests. Suze had made her fortune through fortunate (ex) marriages while Mallory's money came from multiple inheritances. My nest egg was primarily from something laid, not litigated or left to me—a hit erotic film I'd produced in the eighties. Made in the cock market, invested in the stock market, it was the pillow that allowed me to sleep at night.

I had no food or water after midnight and reported for cataract surgery the next morning. For 45 minutes, a bright orange light shined in my eye while a third year resident utilized an ultrasonic device. He extracted the cataract, implanted an artificial lens and all the while a more experienced doctor was teaching him how to perform. "Now go under. Now go over," I heard several times, as if someone was giving knitting lessons.

"Wow, this is a big one," the young resident had said under his breath as he operated. While removing my bandage the next morning, he exclaimed: "I can't believe how much chopping I did on you!" Reading a few eye charts demonstrated accurate vision at a foot away—but with a very noticeable gray film over the affected eye. I still had the macular pucker. "No stooping, lifting or carrying for a month now," he warned, while handing me some aftercare literature.

I had just enough time to recover before The North East Littles conference. How could I resist attending a convention of Adult Babies? And why would I want to spend a weekend with a bunch of diaper wearers? It all began when I met a certain strange but desirable man who lived not too far away.

NINE

Adventures In Babysitting

MY PARENTS HAD TAUGHT ME TO RESPECT military personnel. If I addressed a sailor or soldier when I was a teenager, failure to utter some version of "thank you for your service" resulted in Mother's sharp elbow at my ribcage. My father had been a much-decorated war hero, having rescued several wounded soldiers under heavy fire. He received the Silver Star Medal, the Bronze Star (for a separate act of heroism), the Purple Heart and many pieces of shrapnel in the butt for his efforts.

That's why I was more than positive when a retired military man, Matt*, contacted me. Though he lived in a suburban town filled with churches and cute Victorian homes on tree-lined streets, Matt was not a typical suburbanite. He had no wife or kids (he'd never married) and didn't commute to his Manhattan high-rise office. A man in his fifties, he'd been an officer with a lengthy tour of duty either in Iraq or Afghanistan (I've forgotten which) and the world-weary confidence that came with it. Matt was not eager to be of service to a domme—a military career had been more than enough service for him. Nor did he encourage having more stress or punishment in his life, so he wasn't into BDSM. Now the beneficiary of a decent military service pension plus a sizable parental inheritance, Matt only wanted to be taken care of. He finally had the time and resources to live his dream—being a full-time Adult Baby. But for such a fantasy to be realized, one needs to find a very understanding Mommy.

When we met for a drink, which afterwards became dinner, Matt opened up to me. Aside from his unusual lifestyle aspirations, he was very sure of himself and certain in his goal—to live as an Adult Baby within the confines of his comfortable home. Like most vanilla men I've dated, he was interviewing me for a job. "Can you see yourself changing me in an adult diaper? Would you find any fulfillment cradling me in your arms? Will you let me play with my toys for hours on end uninterrupted, with no adult responsibilities? Could you always address me as a mommy would talk to her baby and never as an adult?"

I actually entertained this strange notion, as good looking Matt comported himself with an appealing quiet strength and dignity. But how could someone with a military background, who seemed so outwardly masculine, spend his days pretending to be a baby? And I had no idea whether I could fill his Mommy role as I'd never before dealt with an Adult Baby. (The fellow who proposed meeting me in public while wearing a diaper outside his clothes was not an Adult Baby but an exhibitionist. Adult Babies keep themselves totally closeted.)

Matt filled me in about an upcoming convention where I would meet many "Littles" (as he noted they were called) and get some hands-on experience. He believed after attending such an affair, I'd know whether a relationship with him could proceed. Though I was initially hesitant, the deal was sealed when he declared: "I'm looking for an older woman." Compared to all the guys I'd met who couldn't date young enough (desiring females the approximate age of their daughters) this Adult Baby seemed a reasonable bet.

That is why I found myself riding the rails to yet another kinkfest in suburban New Jersey. Once I arrived, I was given a choice of color-coded ribbon. "It's yellow if you want to be changed or purple if you're a Mommy and will change others," advised Mike*, who worked security. He required a passport or driver's license to check my age—no one under 21 was allowed to register at NELicon, a yearly get together for the Northeast Littles. On the wall, a large banner bore the NEL logo—an initial N, E and L on three separate sides of a juvenile alphabet block and CON similarly shown on a second block. The Northeast Littles Invasion, read the banner alongside the group's slogan, which proclaimed: We Do Exist!!!

A Little is a kinky adult who engages in age play. Though they get satisfaction pretending to be a baby or child, a Little would never interact this way with actual children, as they are not pedophiles. Parties and conferences are arranged for Littles to be with one another. Most enjoy wearing and wetting diapers plus getting their nappies changed by those they call Mommies and Daddies.

I chose the purple ribbon to wear around my wrist and was given a blank name tag on which I wrote Mommy Joyce. "Oh, you're a Mommy. Great. We've got dozens of ABs and DLs but we need more Bigs," Mike explained. An AB (or Adult Baby) will act as a baby and wear visible diapers but DLs (or Diaper Lovers) like to don their diapers under regular clothes, never appearing or acting as a young child. Then there are ATs or Adult Toddlers, who prefer wearing diapers under overalls or footed sleepers. ATs are more active—they walk instead of crawl and don't see themselves as helpless infants. For adults who imagine themselves as older children (preteens) I've heard the term Middles and also Bedwetters. I wondered whether military man Matt was an AB, a DL or an AT.

Perusing the NELicon schedule, I noticed there were different rooms and events for ABs and DLs. Where Diaper Lovers had discussion groups about their lifestyle and Diaper Modification workshops, the Adult Babies playroom had scheduled activities which included Play With Goo, Coloring Contest, Bubbles Blowing, Cuddles, Nap Time, Games With Mommy, Story Hour, Silly Songs and Play-Doh Making. Diaper Lovers don't behave as young children—they would rather play Wii games while lolling about wetting their diapers.

I asked where most attendees came from. "The North East Littles are mainly people who used to be with SIDNEY," noted Taffy*, a heterosexual married man with children who cross-dressed as a little girl and wore diapers.

"Who is *Sidney?*"

"It's a group and stands for Still In Diapers New York. But SIDNY is now defunct and NEL is taking its place, just as *Diaper Pail Friends* is no longer online but there's *Diaper Tube* and others." (Among them are *Daily Diapers*, *Diaper Space*, and *Adult Baby World*.)

Diaper wearers feel they are deeply misunderstood, necessitating a heavy online presence where they can make contact with others. Groups of like-minded diaper devotees have popped up all over America including CAP (Chicago Age Players) plus more organized Littles chapters in Maryland, Connecticut, Illinois and Pennsylvania.

Adult Babies also have a difficult time finding caregivers, which is why professional mommies exist. Nanny Bliss, based in the Washington, D.C. area, was not at NELicon but Mommy Molly* had come all the way from the Midwest. While pro-dommes in New York City earn upward of $350 an hour, Mommy Molly charged $200 an hour. She even offered a $2,500 cut-rate weekend package deal—and if her expenses were paid, she'd travel to the Adult Baby.

The sweet-tempered but no-nonsense Molly was overweight and extremely self-possessed. When she was not tending to her dozen regular clients (most of whom were married and had hidden this secret life from their spouses) she was a student. She enjoyed a normal romantic and sexual relationship with her boyfriend, who knew what Molly did for a living and grudgingly accepted it.

Mommy Molly made sure no Adult Babies wasted her time, as many men have babyhood fantasies they never act on. She charged men just to talk to her—and they paid even more when making plans to meet. That way, if the potential client backed out, she was covered. "It's a need and I'm providing a service. The guys will tell you what they crave—to be held, spanked, sung to or have their diapers changed." Mommy Molly was acknowledged to be the top pro-mom in adult babydom because of her decade-long experience.

Molly had cut her hourly rate in half for NELicon. A card she handed out explained What Mommy Does In A Session and went on to list (according to client preference and available time) "diaper changes, bath time, playing with toys, baby food feeding, sippy cups and bottles, pacifiers, cartoons, cuddling, spanking and corner time."

Besides Molly and me, there was only one other mommy among the 60 attendees—Mommy Jen*. She came with the fiftyish man she lived with, Baby Jerry*. Jen had first encountered Jerry in one of the many online diaper groups; they had corresponded for two years before meeting. Jerry, who no longer worked, lived off his parents' trust fund. The Florida-based Jen had no place to live when her roommate made her vacate. That's when she moved her belongings to live with Jerry in another state, and be his Mommy. Although they'd never met before cohabitation, Jerry and Jen seemed compatible as any other couple. Mommy Jen summed up why their relationship worked: "Jerry doesn't want a wife or a lover. He wants a mommy and that's what I am to him."

Was this the role military man Matt hoped to play with me? Baby Jerry acted convincingly infantile and showed me his favorite plush toy, a donkey. He'd taken an infant changing blanket and fashioned it into a diaper for the toy, confiding how he carried the diaper-clad donkey everywhere.

NELicon was held at one of the many chain hotels located in New York City's suburbs. Participants were expected to register by Friday and spend two nights on premises. (This lodging establishment had been informed the conference concerned nurturing.) NELicon had booked several meeting rooms to meet attendees' various needs—there was a designated Adult Baby Nursery, Littles Playroom and The Polite DL Lounge. *Polite*, in this context, meant you can wet but not soil your diaper.

As I waited for the elevator on Saturday morning, a heavyset man in his late thirties stood beside me. I noticed he had wrapped a yellow ribbon around his thick wrist and was staring at my purple ribbon. "Would you like to change me?" His manner was sweet and submissive.

"I'm here to learn. I've never changed a diaper before. I don't have kids and only know how to change a litter box."

He called himself Baby Chippy* and didn't push but shyly suggested he could show me how, if I would be his Mommy. After I agreed, we walked to room 111, designated as the Adult Baby Nursery, where the man had stashed his supplies.

Baby Chippy soon doffed all his clothes except for an adult-size diaper worn beneath his size XXL plastic pants—a pair with *b-a-b-y* spelled out on alphabet blocks. He could have gotten them at Plastics & Pinafores, Big Baby Boutique, AB Universe, Bambino or any of the dozen or so American-based businesses which sold clothing and accessories to Adult Babies. Had Baby Chippy gone to Germany or Japan, where adult diapers are really happening, he would have had a far wider choice at several brick and mortar Adult Baby retail stores.

Chippy liked to lie on his back, chubby legs in the air, kicking back and forth a bit. When he didn't have a pacifier in his mouth, he'd suck on a baby bottle filled with a milky substance. I had put his balding head in my lap. Baby Chippy gurgled and clapped his huge hands. Looking back and up at me with wide, faux-innocent eyes, he reached toward my breasts. I was wearing a blouse and sweater over a bra but he just touched the surface of my clothes lightly. He was not an aggressive grabber.

He requested a lullaby and although I didn't know any, I adapted a song from my youth—"My Girl" became "My Mommy." Half way through the song, when I'd begun to forget the lyrics, his mind was on something else. "Can baby have some mommy milk?"

"Mommy is too old to have any milk for baby. For that, you need a young mommy like Mommy Molly, who is a couple hundred dollars an hour."

"So, how can you be a mommy?" his attitude was brattier but still juvenile.

"I froze my eggs."

"Oh. Does baby have potty privileges?" Chippy pushed.

"Tell me more about what that is," I prodded, not entirely understanding.

Every man has a beef about his past girlfriend. But for Chip it wasn't cheating, nagging or overspending. "I used to have a mommy who took away my potty privileges. Then she wouldn't come home when she said she would—she'd make me wait for her with poopy diapers," he recalled in a childlike way. "Some mommies change poopy diapers and others don't—they send baby into the bathroom to shower it off. Which kind of mommy are you?"

"The throw baby out in the street kind." I replied evenly. Baby Chippy was pressing his luck. The North East Littles had sent several messages (to potential conference goers and paid registrants alike) stating there will be absolutely no "number two" allowed, though wetting was permitted.

He continued to speak of his ex-mommy in a babyish falsetto as I looked down at him, stroking his forehead. "She tried to take away my manhood by forcing me to jerk off five times a day. Five times is too, too much and soon I was so worn out I couldn't get hard. I was like a little baby," he finished sweetly. "If baby came to visit Mommy one weekend, could baby bring his play pen and big crib to Mommy's place?"

I'd seen the online sites like *AB Wonders* which sold adult-size baby furniture. "Why do you have to haul in all that stuff? What do you have in mind, Baby Chippy?"

"When you put baby into a crib or playpen, mommy can put up the sides that go high so I'm locked in and can't get out." I later learned how many Adult Babies seek to be controlled. They hate having to make choices; baby play is an escape from having any responsibility. But men with fetishes seldom have just one kink. Chip was an exhibitionist and one who sought humiliation. "If I promise to be a good baby, would you change my diaper in front of a bunch of your girlfriends? I'll come to see you one weekend, and then they could all stand around my crib and poke fun at the big baby."

The guy was seriously hatching plans for a future scene. "Sorry, Baby Chippy, my co-op requires a $500 deposit for moving in furniture and it's Monday to Friday only—you can't bring anything big, like a crib, in on weekends."

"I wet my diaper," he whispered. "Mommy, will you change me?"

Perhaps it was for such occasions the expression *go with the flow* was invented. Baby Chippy plunged the pacifier back in his mouth and reached for a changing pad he'd placed nearby. It had a layer of plastic between the soft cotton coating—he smiled when he heard the familiar crinkle. (I had heard the sound of plastic baby goods being handled is a reassuring one, a turn on for Adult Babies.) I placed this beneath his big bulk, pulled off the protective plastic pants, and removed his wet diaper, which he tossed into a conveniently placed diaper pail.

He spread apart his chubby thighs, exposing his clean-shaven, flaccid genitals and told me his baby wipes were in a nearby duffle bag. I could see traces of powder as I cleaned up around his testicles. He asked for more talcum, handing me a bottle of Johnson's Baby Powder, which I sprinkled on his sex organs like powdered sugar on a soft croissant. He then pointed to the fresh paper diaper and raised his bottom so it could be placed beneath him.

Once I'd figured out which part of the diaper went over and up, and found the adhesive tabs, I thought I was home free. But before I could secure the diaper on each side, Chippy begged, in an even more babyish voice, if he could "make creamy."

He first squirted some baby lotion down there and without any tactile help from me, the man cooed and gurgled as he happily masturbated. (After giving him permission to use lotion, I'd removed myself from the bed.) It didn't take Chip long to come, lying there with the unfastened diaper beneath him. When he motioned for me to pull the adhesive tabs and diaper him, I suggested he use a baby wipe first. "No, the diaper will absorb all that," Chip replied in an adult tone, as if the baby act had finished with his orgasm. I asked myself whether this sort of thing was what Matt expected.

I saw Chippy a few hours later in the Littles Playroom wearing a baby blue onesie, crawling on the carpet while clutching a plush toy to his beefy neck and sucking on a pacifier. Joining him there were six other guys. One wore a long sleeper with a back flap, another had donned short denim overalls on top of a pastel, short sleeved t-shirt. NELicon attendees were often warned not to wear their baby gear, carry their teddy bears or show their diapers in the hotel lobby—all kiddie garb and activities were on the down-low. While a praise-the-Lord type church group prayed in the meeting room across the hall, in the Littles

Playroom, over a dozen adults were dressed either as young children or babies, with an even number of boys to girls. According to the *Daily Diapers* website, there's a male-female split of 60/40 among diaper wearers, roughly the same as at NELicon.

Of the seven men in the playroom, three were cross-dressed as girls. Taffy was a forty-something guy wearing black Mary Jane shoes with white socks and a short pinafore printed in a cartoon rabbit motif. A blonde pigtailed wig completed the effect. The sixtyish Baby David wore an even shorter frilly dress with a white baby bonnet, meant to represent an infant baby girl. Most Littles were sprawled on the floor face down using crayons and coloring books, or sitting up on their knees building with Tonka toys. A man and woman, each dressed as a baby boy or girl, both sucked on special adult-sized pacifiers and giggled as they beat each other with green foam rubber bats shaped like swords.

I ran into Mommy Molly in the hall. "Molly, is it normal for male babies to ask for your milk?"

"Yes, very, but I do no breastfeeding. It's actually illegal in some locations."

"And is it typical for an AB guy to masturbate before being diapered?"

"Yes, but I won't have any of it. It's sexual contact. Not allowed. You can use the Schick Quattro shaver on them if they like being smooth down there but no yanking," she counseled briskly, patting me on the shoulder before waddling away.

Molly and I were recruited to supervise the Saturday afternoon Games With Mommy held in the Littles Playroom. She knew just how to lead the group into a game of Mommy Says and we took turns ordering the dozen plus Littles into different Simon Says scenarios. I observed how several name tags bore the suffix *chan*. A cross-dressing fellow in his twenties was a hyphen *chan* as were two girls in their early twenties.

"Why do so many Adult Babies have *chan* after their names?" I asked Taffy. It was early Saturday evening and we were watching the Adult Baby Fashion show. Several Littles walked a makeshift runway to loud nursery-appropriate tunes and enthusiastic applause. (A vendor supplied the colorful, comfy clothes. Later at the Los Ninos Tex-Mex dinner, winning models were announced.) "*Chan* means adorable little girl in Japanese," Taffy explained. "The twenty-somethings or college kids came to wearing diapers through the Japanese anime culture that's such a big influence over here."

One such college girl, Lori-chan*, approached us. "Will you help me pin my bow?" she requested in a dulcet child's tone. Her navy blue private school uniform was pure Cosplay, a term derived from costume play, which was largely inspired by Japanese anime, cartoons or video games. I pinned her red bow to a prim white cotton blouse worn beneath a tailored dark blue jacket, one bearing a school logo patch over the breast pocket. A matching kilt with white knee-high socks completed the Japanese schoolgirl look.

I had known how Japanese are big on *kwai* or cuteness, which finds expression in anime characters, plush toys, Hello Kitty accessories and kiddie fashions. But diapers? "Since where are diapers *kwai?*" I asked Taffy.

"Oh, diapers are very *kwai*, very big with the youth culture. If you don't believe me, google Japanese anime and diapers."

After dinner I used the hotel computer to do as Taffy suggested, and almost immediately, dozens of images appeared. The cartoons featured uniformed schoolgirls with their legs apart, a yellow stain spread on their exposed diapers, and a helpless look on those oversized faces. They typically featured big eyes and a smaller mouth—the proportions found on a baby, which we visually interpret as a state of innocence. But it was not just young girls long past their potty training years who were depicted as diapered, and using pacifiers or sucking on a baby bottle. I viewed infantilized and diapered preteen boys with non-diapered adult males. They often appeared alongside popular anime characters like Pokemon's Pikachu, who had been spared the diaper. I found no images of solid waste on diapers, nothing depicting sexual conduct and very little showing diapers on those who actually wear them—babies and toddlers.

Before I could find Taffy to tell him he was right, I ran into one of the NELicon organizers. "You're one of the few Mommies attending. We're auctioning off an hour session with Mommy Molly for Sunday morning. Would you be the other Mommy people can bid on?"

"Jeez, I just diapered my first AB today. I'm not so sure I know what I'm doing, as Mommy Molly does."

"Oh, you'll be fine," he assured me. "There'll be a big interest in being with Mommy Joyce. And it's for a good cause."

I encountered Taffy in the hallway outside the Little Rascals Theater. In public spaces such as the hotel hall, he'd stash his blonde wig in a bag and put a raincoat over his pinafore. Although Taffy was handsome with a conservative appearance, in the way of a news anchor, he still looked like a flasher. Taffy pulled me aside to report: "Lori-chan is going to wet her first diaper but she's a little anxious about it. So she wants a woman there. Will you change her?"

"I don't deal with women," I answered dismissively, before adding: "And I certainly don't have enough experience."

"O.K.," he answered easily. "I'll recruit Mommy Molly."

Doing diaper duty on a girl, especially one young enough to be my daughter, simply creeped me out. But the next morning, it should have come as no surprise when I was told the winning bid for Mommy Joyce's nurturing hour was from a college-aged girl.

I'd seen the petite brunette Rikki-chan* napping on a blankie, sucking on her pacifier and making Play-Doh animals when I supervised the Littles Playroom. "How old are you?" I asked as she confidently led me to her hotel room.

"About one and a half. I can't speak yet." For either her fantasy age or her biological age, she was far more poised and in control than I, at over sixty.

"O.K., but I've got to tell you—I've only taken care of one Adult Baby before and it went down yesterday. I fed him his bottle, changed his diapers. Do you like all that?"

"Yes, please. Plus baby food and a bath. And some cuddles." She spoke as an adult.

"Do you like guys or girls?"

"I'm not gay just because I want a mommy to take care of me. In real life, who takes care of babies? The mommies. All the daddies I've met who are into diapering girls—they get off on diapers with *sex*," she confided, wrinkling her pert little nose. "I'm into wearing diapers, being taken care of, and getting babied—but not diaper sex. That's all so *not me,* and just so *not* what this is all about. It's an experience of being nurtured, going back to a pleasant time in my life. It's what I like and makes me feel good."

After turning on the bath water, I visualized military man Matt within his cozy suburban home. Was this what he was looking for? I began to undress my young charge as she passively lay on the hotel bed. "Lift your hips, little baby." Rikki-chan gurgled and cooed as I struggled with her tight spandex jeans and undid her bra. Now completely nude and affecting helplessness, she leaned on me. I offered my arm as she walked with unsteady legs to her bath.

Rikki-chan uttered some unbelievably authentic sounding baby noises while splashing about in the tub. Her pubic hair was natural and untrimmed, the breasts full as well. The most unusual thing about her naked body was the sizable Japanese anime character which had been tattooed in a noticeable spot. I soaped up a washcloth and began scrubbing her arms, legs, torso and back as she closed her eyes and smiled, sometimes hitting the bathwater surface with her open hands and squealing in joy. I had heard about diaper lovers entering "baby bliss" as they regressed, and thought this was what she was experiencing.

I got her to stand up, helped her out of the tub, then towel-dried the girl before leading her back to the bed. Her gait was as wobbly as before. I first put the diaper pad down on the mattress before having her lie down and lift her legs, which she kicked back and forth a bit in a relaxed rhythm. I fastened one side of the adult diaper with its velcro tabs, then the other. The diaper now on, she squealed with glee and slapped her thighs with the palms of both hands. A short, frilly pink dress with puff sleeves and a full skirt had been placed nearby. I helped her into it, as if she had no prior experience with putting her arms through sleeve holes. Considering the various baby noises Rikki-chan was making, she seemed to be thoroughly enjoying herself.

I cradled my arm for her head and tilted back her baby bottle so she could chug-a-lug Similac while leaning against my chest. Baby formula must be an acquired taste for adults, but she gulped it down hungrily and sucked on the nipple with a regular rhythm as her cheeks hollowed and filled again. While I held the bottle she looked up at me with such a needy expression, I considered perhaps she had been studying acting at school. Could she be authentically experiencing the helplessness of an infant? I held Rikki-chan against my breasts and patted her on the back until I heard her emit some stomach gas.

The girl babbled and pointed to some Gerber baby food in plastic containers she'd placed on a nearby nightstand. A pink terry cloth baby bib lay beside it along with a small-sized, pink plastic-coated metal spoon. I tied the bib around her neck, picked up the spoon, dipped it in the small glass jar and began feeding her as she lay propped up against me and in my arms. "Here comes the choo-choo train," I chirped, having heard this is what mommies tell their progeny before cramming food in their mouths. Rikki-chan opened wide and clapped her hands together, seemingly in delight. I tried not to get any apple-blueberry formula on her baby dress, but she purposely let the food dribble out the sides of her mouth, down her chin and onto the bib because that's where she thought the food should be.

After feeding her, I removed the food-stained bib and popped a jumbo sized pacifier between her lips. (Baby pacifiers are a size two, I learned, while Adult Babies use a size five.) As she held a stuffed animal and sucked away, I sang her old songs as a gentle lullaby, all the while stroking her hands, arms and scalp. I hoped it had been an hour full of gentleness for Rikki-chan while she revealed her inner self to another, a stranger who'd assumed the caregiver role.

It was soon time for the Little Miss Adult Baby Princess Contest, which Rikki-chan was keen to enter. Our session over, we could now speak to each other as adults. I helped her into a short lacy black sateen Gothic Lolita number. (In Cosplay, the term Lolita does not imply sex—Lolitas dress modestly and go for a cutesy yet elegant effect. Gothic Lolitas wear mainly black with a few crosses and other Goth touches in the mix.) As I tied her back sash and buttoned her Peter Pan collar, I laughed about the fact I had a Cosplay outfit, too—I dressed as the anime character Sailor Moon.

Rikki-chan seemed surprised to hear this, as if a teen had learned her Mom had discovered and was secretly listening to Iggy Azalea. "You're kidding? Very cool. I like anything Japanese. Sushi. Kimonos. Toyotas. Are you into anime?"

"No. I just go as a Sailor Moon, the Japanese schoolgirl, on Halloween."

After Rikki-chan went on to win the Little Miss Adult Baby Princess title, Taffy recruited me to help him feed her in a special high chair he'd brought to NELicon. He had taken a plastic car seat meant for special needs children and retrofitted it into a BDSM contraption. Taffy covered Rikki-chan's black sateen smock with a plastic bib and asked if we could secure her hands and feet in restraints. After she nodded a consent, I helped place her wrists and ankles into the velcro closed cuffs which attached to the high chair. Taffy then proposed he put in a pacifier she could not remove. The girl gurgled an agreement then opened her mouth for a forced pacifier, one attached to a strap in back of her head. Rikki-chan took to bondage as enthusiastically as she was into anything Japanese, or being babied.

Taffy, now changed out of his pigtailed wig and pinafore, was kind enough to drive me to the train station. I'd met some people, had new experiences, learned a lot—exactly what you take away from most conferences. But for Taffy, the high point of NELicon was being there on Saturday night for Lori's first wetting.

The 21-year-old Lori-chan had told her parents where she was going (to a Littles convention) and what she would be doing (dressing as a child). She revealed to them her longing—she had felt a desire to wear diapers ever since she was about five years old. (Around age five is when those who later become Adult Babies first feel the urge to get back into diapers for emotional comfort.) Lori's parents didn't understand, she confessed—instead they were horrified.

Taffy had rubbed Lori-chan's feet to make her feel comfortable as she sat in his big high chair. With much trepidation, she'd urinated in a diaper for the very first time, something young Lori had been fantasizing about for several years. Taffy later spoke about the event: "Her candor, sweetness and innocence were all so touching. The way she allowed me to be there—it was such a privilege to be a part of her first wetting," he declared with father-of-the-bride pride and emotion.

As Taffy took my luggage out of his car, a nearby woman observed us, as we appeared to be an attractive couple. Out of his Taffy clothes he looked every bit the middle aged hottie, thoroughly assured and comfortable in his conservative preppy wear. "You've got to get into wearing diapers yourself," he advised me, smiling seductively. "The secret, the crinkle, the wetness. You'll love it."

But taking care of an Adult Baby was not one of the many sensory experiences I was then craving. It just wasn't a desirable 24/7 lifestyle for me, as I later explained to a disappointed Matt. After recovering from years of crippling pain and having turned sixty, I wanted to be taken care of. It was neither mommy-domme nor a vanilla husband I sought. I began to wonder whether it was a submissive man I was looking for, or just maybe a slave.

TEN

When Slavehood Was In Flower

I NEEDED A SUBMISSIVE WHO WASN'T TOO extreme, one who could pass for vanilla, and imagined the local munches (conveniently held in some Chelsea diners nearby) a logical place to meet such a man. Once at the munch, I sat next to Bradley*, a corporate executive in his fifties who lived in New York City's suburbs and worked in Connecticut. Though I found Bradley attractive, he had a decidedly dated look. Dressed as an office park dweller circa 1984, he wore the baby blue Oxford cloth shirt above a pair of pleated baggy khaki pants. On a more positive note, he'd introduced himself as *slave* Bradley. After we'd spoken for a bit, his compliments were effusive. "You are a golden flower in a toxic field of weeds!" The man was ready to worship.

Bradley appeared to regard me as I saw myself. Whether he called himself a submissive or slave, I wanted someone who thought I was a prize, treat me accordingly, and make few (if any) demands. We talked again on the phone before I chose where he could take me for dinner. My wish was his command.

I picked a restaurant on the Upper East Side where I could comfortably nestle into a cushy banquette and peruse my prey. Slave Bradley was punctual and acted the perfect gentleman. He did nothing to embarrass me at the restaurant, unlike Harold*, the chivalry buff I'd dated a month before. I'd agreed to meet Harold because he expressed an interest in knighthood and medieval times. We'd just ordered our drinks before it became apparent Harold's interests were more focused around ghoulish torture devices. I had interrupted him, declaring The Rack, Judas Cradle and the like is hardly dinner conversation, and he should immediately return to discussing chivalry. My criticism had prompted him to abruptly leave his chair, go down on one bended knee, clasp my hand in his and pledge his undying servitude. Witnessing that bit of business spurred those at nearby tables to spontaneously clap and cheer—they thought a marriage proposal was in the offing and I was getting engaged to this kinkster.

I had thought *slave* Bradley, as he always called himself, a perfect mild-mannered milquetoast. A fellow who made a decent appearance, yet could disappear into the woodwork was just my style. Bradley preferred I order for the two of us, claiming it excited him to see me take the dominant role. I noticed how his chest, somewhat expanded by gym membership, puffed up even more when I emphasized to our waiter how my meat must be very rare. Many vanilla men I'd dated liked to order for me. The absolute worst thing I could do when dining out would be to complain about the food—such behavior was viewed as an embarrassment, their date regarded as a neurotic bitch. But when the rare steak I ordered came back cooked as medium, and I sent the meat back because "it's not pink enough inside," my date seemed to reach such a state of ecstasy I thought he'd spill in his chinos. About five years younger than I, his once tender heart was now encrusted with a certain middle aged bitterness.

Bradley was never ambivalent about women. Either he was awestruck in admiration for powerful women he'd never met or he'd rail about the general unsuitability of the women he *did* know and escort. The latter seemed to be all dommes, all the time. He didn't date vanilla women, even if they came on to him. Such enticements were actually frequent, as Bradley had a management position in a lucrative industry. He related his recent rendezvous with a Normal Nancy: "There's a single woman at my office who's really pretty. I ran into her and we started talking about a certain film showing at the local cineplex. We both wanted to see it. But I was so disappointed in how she lacked the initiative to ask me out! She looked at me with such expectation. And I thought—*why can't she just take the bull by the horns and suggest we go to the movies*? I was really turned off by her being so passive. I mean, did she expect *me* to step up to the plate and do the asking? Lately, I've been avoiding even speaking to her—I just turn my head or look the other way." He looked down in disgust before his gaze returned to beam across the table. "But you! I saw the way you handled that waiter!"

"I had just told him how I like my meat really, very rare—and when it came out too cooked inside..."

"Mistress Pussycat," he interrupted, using my scene name in a voice of sheer adulation, "you were magnificent."

A first date is for getting to know each other. During an after dinner stroll, I probed into his earliest childhood memories and boyhood fantasies. Bradley poignantly recalled how his first erotic feelings surfaced—a neighbor girl beat him with a stick in her backyard. When another young female flayed him with a rope, he reached an even greater prepubescent sexual frenzy, and consciously provoked her to ensure more punishment. Watching *Wonder Woman* on TV further fed his masturbatory fantasies. Each night he would lie in his college dorm bed, fondling his penis while imagining Wonder Woman tying him to a tree with her golden lasso, or kicking him with her spurred boots—leaving him struggling, defeated and helpless. Summer-themed teen movies were more masturbatory fodder, especially when a buxom bikinied babe would trample underfoot, kick sand on, or otherwise humiliate some chump on a beach blanket. Glorious, strong gladiator girls were his feminine ideal: when their sandal-shod feet were placed on a hapless male's chest, this victory pose sent Bradley into a paroxysm of joy. Such fantasies would be constant in his mind's automatic re-run loop; but back on Earth, the girls he dated wondered what was missing in such-a-nice-guy. Bradley admitted he was a confused young man and regretted his misguided marriage to a pure vanilla woman, a union which produced the grown daughter who lived nearby. Although he loved his daughter and two toddler grandchildren, Bradley thought of his marriage as a mistake made when he should have known better. Even while he was wed, Bradley realized female domination, and a woman who understood his submissive side, was what he craved.

When we first met, I had told him I was soon going on vacation. At the end of our first date, Bradley asked when he could see me again. I reminded him I was packing and too busy to get together.

"I would like to see you again, before you leave, if possible," he said softly. "Even if it's just to drive you to the airport and carry your bags."

I thanked him and declared it unnecessary, noting how I'd use my usual car service. But the very next day it was unseasonably warm, my co-op hadn't switched the convectors from heat to chill and Best Buy was having a sale on window unit air conditioners. I'd just bought one when Bradley called; I mentioned how someone had to bring the unit back to my place. "I would be honored to handle the pick-up," he replied. "I have kept tomorrow totally free of responsibilities, so I am your slave for the day, if you so desire." As much as I craved being cool, the thought of having a slave man do my bidding gave me a pleasant, warm feeling. But Best Buy would deliver for very little money, I learned, and decided this was easiest.

After returning from Europe, I began to see more of Bradley. He shared with me his favorite kinky website, which he urged me to view. The blog which kept him enthralled was ostensibly written by a psychiatrist who had made a slave of her husband. The kinky shrinky kept her hubby drugged and submissive by the careful, constant administration of psychotropic prescription pharmaceuticals. Each new posting had Bradley cheering for this wife, who coerced her helpless mate to engage in creative deviations. She'd often perform random acts of cruelty on his lanky body. "What'd you think of that blog? Don't you just love her?" he asked on the phone, after I'd seen the wife grinding her shoe's stiletto heel into her husband's nuts, then cross-dressing him.

"I'm not a fan. It's obviously fake and staged. As a femdom role model, I'd rather have a domme who does not exploit her partner."

"I thought you might like it," he said sheepishly.

"I don't mean to seem disapproving; it actually made me laugh. It's kinkster kitsch—so bad it's almost good."

Bradley's other heroine was a recently deceased European dominatrix who'd written a book about the severe brand of discipline she practiced with her two male live-in slaves. "Mistress would give her slave one thrash of the cane for every hair she found on his body," Bradley reverently recounted. For many slaves, being completely hairless is a point of pride—some shave their heads even when blessed with a full head of hair.

Bradley was a walker, as I was. I would stroll the streets of Manhattan taking the lead, with Bradley trailing behind, which was the accepted slave street etiquette and how Prince Phillip walked behind his wife, Queen Elizabeth. Bradley loved to escort me everywhere—even to the hairdresser, while holding my little bag of hair care products in his hand. He'd even offer to carry my purse if it was very full and thought it too heavy for my shoulder. While I was getting my tresses treated or working out, he'd eagerly await my orders to buy granola or pick up a Sunday *Times*.

Though vacuuming was a chore he wholeheartedly embraced, Bradley found his purest bliss helping me with the wash. Each time I firmly reminded him in which chute to put the detergent for prewash, I'd notice a wave of pleasure settle over his face, transforming those delicate WASPy features into the semblance of an aged choirboy. "I love this," he'd murmur as he poured the Tide.

"What is it you love about doing laundry?"

"I love the whole role reversal."

Though I was fascinated by Bradley, I had no sexual interest in him. But there was very little work for mother here. He demanded no dramatics, testicle wreckage, doggie walks, not even so much as a whack on the back. Bradley was one easy going sub. And at 61 years of age, I was happy to be waited on and worshipped. Though the sexual attraction was strictly one-sided, I was gratified to get a good massage. I never fully disrobed and he often concentrated on just my feet—yet these massages were an intense erotic experience for him. If I had requested a vanilla man rub my veiny, corn-riddled feet until I fell asleep and never even touched him in return, I'm sure I would have seen the last of him. But slave Bradley told me how he viewed such selfish behavior: "I've never stroked a woman's feet for over an hour. I really loved how you so freely moaned and purred. You're not afraid to show your pleasure, to demand your contentment, which is the ultimate aphrodisiac."

He preferred for me to plan our activities and also let me set the pace sexually—a snail's pace. No, as snails are sexually active hermaphrodites, it was actually the pace of a neutered snail. I had been dating Bradley for nearly three months before I even saw him stroke himself. One night, I came out of my bathroom wearing blue spandex lingerie then lay down on the bedroom quilt. Bradley was encouraged to masturbate while standing by the bed. He looked, unzipped, jerked, then spent some seed in his cupped hand as I heard a low, satisfied growl escape his throat. His erection was strong and sizable, the time to come completely average. Bradley confessed it was one of the most intense orgasms he'd ever had. I'd briefly contemplated clasping his stiffie between the soles of my feet and jerking him off in this manner, but decided it would be a bit too intimate.

His way was best for Bradley, who expressed his satisfaction during a phone call the next day. "I think I had the most sensual moment of my life last night. You showed such confidence and trust. I don't know how you do it, but every time we meet, you empty your quiver into my heart. And it's the bullseye every time."

For the first three months we saw each other, he would never suggest spending the night together—instead he'd drive back to his suburban home. "You know how much I want to stay overnight with you, Mistress Pussycat. But I'm leaving just to prove my intentions are honorable. I am a relationship person, and want to make sure you know that about me through actions, not just words." After we'd been seeing each other for more than three months, he would stay over but never sleep in my bed. He preferred slumbering alone on my living room couch. As he explained during a weekday phone call: "There is too much sexual tension for me between your sheets. Besides, I'd never have fallen asleep anyway. I would have lain there caressing your back and shoulders all night long. I wish we were together right now, my arm around your tiny waist. You have shoulders to die for, so soft and round, made to be caressed. I'd love to smother those shoulders with kisses."

He'd often declare my shoulders were his favorite spot on my anatomy. While there's nothing odd about a man admiring a certain body part, Bradley never made a single move to put his arm around my waist or kiss the shoulders he claimed to adore. As for the actual object of his desire, I had fairly frail shoulders above a prominent ribcage and collarbone in front, with defined vertebrae in back. He made no mention of, and never even touched, the big bouncy breasts that were my better body assets.

Presenting as an attractive, normal heterosexual male, Bradley had left quite a few perplexed women in his wake. By the time we met, he had been exclusively seeking the company of dommes and claimed to have just broken up with one he'd been seeing for years. In the beginning of our courtship, he referred to her as "my old domme" (as if I were his new domme). His attitude towards her was a mixture of respect, sympathy and disgust. He was proud she was, he claimed, a medical doctor and at the same time, a pro-domme. His loathing was provoked because she never cleaned after herself, kept a filthy house and relied on him to do her housework. Yet his sympathy was also triggered by her chronic, increased loss of kidney function. More dialysis would not work—she'd confided in him she would die within a year. He called her Doctor Domme* and though he swore he was repelled by her, he was clearly in awe.

Because she was well versed in health and nutrition, he was forever quoting her wisdom. "Doctor Domme says never eat cooked macadamia nuts as the hot oil harms the nutrients, so only consume them dry roasted or raw." If we passed a fruit stand, Bradley would look at the grapes and remark how Doctor Domme would never eat grapes from outside of the United States and avoided unregulated and excessive use of pesticides.

"She sounds like a PhD maybe, but not a medical doctor."

"No, she is a real doctor. That much I know!" he was adamant. "She's very well educated and accomplished! Why put the lady down?"

"It's just hard to believe a physician is also a practicing dominatrix who does paid sessions. What's her specialty?"

"She specializes in medical play," he explained with a look of pride. "She wears all whites, has all the equipment, the training, knowledge and skills."

"I mean what area of medicine does she specialize in? Where is her office? She's affiliated with which hospital?"

"Oh, I don't know if she goes into the office or makes regular hospital rounds anymore, she's way too infirm now. But she is a real medical doctor and the top dominatrix in the tri-state area who specializes in medical play."

He'd often brag about her recent activities. One of her clients was an adult man with a very successful career whose testicles had never descended. For this reason, Bradley explained, the guy paid Doctor Domme lavish fees to torture his penis with electrical instruments of various voltages, and other devices called sharps. According to Bradley, Doctor Domme referred to this tragic testicular-free fellow as a *fully functioning defective*. "But she's careful," Bradley remarked, "and knows what she's doing because she's a doctor." No Jewish mother was ever more proud of her son the doctor than this submissive man was of his Doctor Domme.

Doctor Domme's domicile didn't sound too sanitary—not from Bradley's description of her mildewed shower stall, the crud in her toilet bowl, and vermin crawling on her unwashed dishes. "She needs me," he'd whimper in a tone of compassion mixed with a tinge of revulsion. "She can't tidy up on her own because she's too weak."

About once a month, always on a Sunday, Bradley would ask my permission if he could go over to Doctor Domme's and clean for her. I always said it was fine, as there's a code of honor between dommes—one always helps another. On Bradley's return, he'd bitterly complain about her, telling me the place was so filthy he ran through five pairs of rubber gloves, and on several occasions nearly heaved. I asked him why he performed these tasks if they revolted him so.

"Because if I didn't do it for her, it would never get done," he sighed. He'd soon after brag about some medical play business she'd recently performed on a paying sub.

"How could she do such a thing when I thought she was too weak to clean?"

"Oh, she's way too physically deteriorated to mop and scrub but it doesn't take any strength to do a catheter. It takes skill and medical knowledge."

He didn't encourage any sexual contact between us, but was happiest wiping down my glass topped dining table or kitchen counter. Scrubbing my bathtub made him feel especially fulfilled. Bradley was your basic service bottom and cleaning for anyone who he thought was a superior woman turned him on.

Then there was the other ex. He often spoke of a domme named Goddess Gina*. "I call a dominant woman *mistress* until she's had a child and then she is a *goddess* if she has..." He paused for dramatic effect. "Created life," he continued in a hushed voice.

Gina, a goddess two times over, had recently put a restraining order on one of the life forms she created, a thuggish 22-year-old daughter who'd taken a swing at Gina and knocked out some front teeth. Bradley described Gina's daughter as a mentally unstable alcoholic. He then explained she was the good child, as Goddess Gina's older, drug addict son was even more of a brute.

According to Bradley, Goddess Gina had raised her teenagers alone while working from home as a pro-domme. When the kids rebelled, she thought it was entirely her fault they were so screwed up. Bradley agreed. "They're lashing out at their Mom and venting anger because of what had gone on in the house." Goddess Gina had only recently hung up her electric cattle prod and leather garter belt, retiring from full-time domination. She now lived on disability. "She just can't seem to get her life together," Bradley would mutter, shaking his head. "She's trouble."

Such sentiments did not keep him away from Goddess Gina's lair. Every other week he'd ask to visit either Doctor Domme or Goddess

Gina and sort out some domestic problem—clean or do chores. "I know you own me, Mistress Pussycat, but my old domme who is dying wants to see her hometown for the last time in her life. She needs me to drive her down for this final sentimental journey. And since chivalry is my personal code, I would consent only if you deem it wise and grant me your permission." Then there was Goddess Gina's cat which was constantly in heat. "Mistress, the Goddess Gina beseeched me to enquire if you could possibly lend me out for a day. Her cat needs to get spayed. I should drive them to the ASPCA on Saturday and pay for it to be done. Gina never gets her life in order and it's not fair the cat has to suffer for it. But I will abide by your decision. My weekends are yours until you tell me otherwise."

Of course, I gave the O.K. to get the cat spayed. I also agreed my slave should take the dying Doctor Domme for a day of suburban-side grave shopping. But I hardly swallowed his stories, remembering he'd mentioned weeks before Gina's cat was a 12-year-old male. This devoted sub who called himself a slave was a first-rate run around Ricky, but one who asked permission first before playing with others. "You get the final say, Mistress Pussycat, because you own me. Your wants, needs and desires come before mine. The only time I am really free is when I'm with you. Because being a woman's slave is who I am deep inside."

I'd dated many a player. But when keeping company with a man who insists you actually *own* him, invoking the fidelity concept seemed complicated, even ridiculous. Prior to Bradley, I had known submissive men—yet now realized those who identified as slaves were different. The ownership concept is specific to slaves, not subs. Although many slaves are lawfully married to their masters (or mistresses), when a slave is *owned* there is a written contract and often a collaring ceremony. Although people in the lifestyle take ownership as seriously as marriage, it's just another form of intimate commitment meant to be binding between two people. Bradley was in no way owned by me—he just called himself a slave and considered himself owned because it turned him on.

I was actually relieved to let slave Bradley clean Doctor Domme's toilet or take Goddess Gina to her local healthcare clinic—I was seeing other submissive men at the same time. Not only did Bradley know about it, the idea excited him. One sub took me to a Broadway matinee (*The Book of Mormon* was in previews) and to dinner after the theater. I told Bradley I would not be available that Saturday.

"I don't want to interfere with your plans," he responded. "But I'd love to come over and tidy up for you on Saturday morning, then help you get ready for your date. You know how I love to be teased!"

I also knew how many submissive men love to be cuckolded. And I was being constantly compared to Bradley's two professional play partners. My apartment was not a challenge to clean, as was Doctor Domme's. "Oh, she's a pro-domme and the minute I walk in her front door, I have to fall on my knees and kiss her ass," he confided. "Then she puts me in my apron."

I remembered how, some 30 years ago, I had tried to beef up my sex performance—I was dating men I met through business, men who also bedded porn stars. Decades later, while seeing submissive men, I similarly felt the need to compete. For this reason, I gave Bradley the list of slave positions I'd previously used with Denny Vinny. Bradley was to assume these postures on my command, unless I instructed him to be at ease. There must be some ritual to differentiate between femdom and vanilla relationships, I decided. I sent him the positions:

*PRESENT *stand or kneel, remove clothes, cross wrists behind back, eyes lowered*

*RESTRICT *cross wrists behind back*

*REST *Sit on heels, legs spread and hands palms up on top of legs*

*SUBMIT *Sit on heels, lean forward until head touches ground. Place arms overhead with palms up and wrists crossed.*

I was anxious to see his reaction. The next time Bradley entered my front door, his head was already bowed in submission. Gone was his usual greeting and wide-eyed appreciative look, taking me in from head to heels. He'd traded in his happy-to-be-here smile for a more solemn demeanor. "Present!" I commanded him sternly.

He immediately shed his clothes, got down on both knees and crossed his wrists behind his back. After spontaneously placing a kiss on one of my bare feet, Bradley trained his eyes on the rug. I grabbed the rhinestone-studded leather dog collar and fastened it about his neck. “Oh, Mistress!”

“Silence!” I snarled, while walking around him, taking pleasure in the sight of a naked Bradley, his head hanging and encircled by the collar. Not only did the collar and submissive stance improve his overall appearance, I found it appealing. Was this collar and kneeling ritual meaningful to him in any way? I had to ask.

“Rise,” I ordered, before instructing him to be at ease. “You may begin regular conversation with me now.” A naked Bradley was standing upright but still fixated on the floor. “You can look ahead, it’s all right.” I was feeling pretty pleased with myself, as if we’d made this huge advancement in our relationship. “Did you like assuming the slave positions?”

“Yes, Mistress Pussycat.”

“Does Goddess Gina make you do anything similar?”

“Oh, yes, Mistress. She has me get down on all fours to be her furniture, but she’s a smoker so she mainly likes me to serve as her human ashtray. ”

“I find that rather harsh. I’m not a smoker and don’t like sitting on anything too hard. At least I don’t make you kiss my ass, like when you walk into Doctor Domme’s.”

“You don’t make me drink a cup of her piss on entering, either.”

“What? You say you *drink her urine*? I don’t believe this!”

“Sure. It’s another ritual, like she’s marking me. Animals mark their territory with their urine. Besides, pee is pretty pure stuff. If you run out of water and you’re in the desert, you can drink your piss. It’s not like she’s making me consume any solid waste.”

“But didn’t you tell me she has less than a year left due to failing kidney function? And don’t the kidneys filter toxins out of the urine? How could a dying doctor allow you to drink her poisonous waste matter, especially if you say she’s so fucking health conscious?” Although I was screeching, his voice was low and level, meant to placate me.

“Hey, don’t freak out. I’ve been drinking it for years and it hasn’t killed me yet. Don't worry—I'm in the hands of a medical doctor."

I was relieved to realize I'd never even kissed him. As we left my apartment, I reminded myself to contact slave Ralph*, a fellow in his early fifties, who'd been recommended to me by another domme. Ralph had emphasized he wanted only one mistress. Though he had provided little information about himself, I thought maybe he'd be more my style—or at the very least, have a little more sense.

Ralph was only available to speak after nine p.m. at the number he'd provided. Unlike other submissive men I'd interviewed on the phone, he was unguarded, almost guileless. I had a million questions for him, and he answered every one with a quiet sincerity. Ralph tried to fill me in about his life as best as he could, considering he did not really know who he was.

He was certain his name was Ralph but was confused about his last name, his parents and identity. He recalled not being permitted to attend school after third grade and believed he was from West Virginia, but wasn't really sure as he was sold into slavery at the age of eight. "I always remember myself as a slave and can't recall a time when I was not owned." Ralph had worked as a slave to one family until he'd turned 17, when he was again sold, this time to a much older woman. "That owner was very strict. She liked to hurt me and I was always kept in the house. I wasn't ever allowed outdoors." After several years, he was once more sold, now to a young prostitute, who he described as the most beautiful woman he'd ever seen. As Ralph related how he had never been permitted to watch TV, read the newspaper, or go outside of where he resided, he had little basis for comparison.

It was fascinating to hear how he felt about her, their association, on being a slave. "When I am a lady's slave, it's like I become a part of her. I like knowing I am important to my owner and I enjoy being used."

"Did you enjoy being hurt by her?"

"No, I don't like pain, not at all. But I know she did those things out of love, which is why I submit. Love is very important to me. I don't really look at it as pain because anything that comes from my owner is divine."

"You say you enjoy being used. Do you mean working and serving or used some other way?"

Besides doing household duties, Ralph also pleasured women during the many sex parties his mistress held. These slutty soirees were attended by both men and women—all participants paid Ralph's mistress serious money to satisfy their wildest fantasies. There he performed oral sex on women and gave sexual massages. "My penis was not to be used," Ralph confessed, before detailing how it had been placed into a chastity device.

Did he know how female enforced chastity was a method for lowering testosterone and controlling males? "Why do you think she put away your penis?"

"I don't know. But my owner always had my best interests at heart," he declared.

I asked how he felt being used as a party toy. "If someone was to use me for sex, I was told what I would be doing and how I was to be used." He didn't believe he'd been abused in any way.

Ralph enjoyed the many books he was permitted to read, mainly classics, and could write. He knew the name of the street he had lived on, realized they had resided in Queens, but was unsure of his last name as he had no birth certificate or Social Security card.

When answering my questions about the former owner, Ralph became more hesitant. That part of his story came out in pieces and only after my incessant prodding, as if it was unthinkable not to obey my orders. But when the talk was unrelated to this woman, he responded with a sense of serenity and acceptance, freely explaining his background and intimate aspects of his life. Ralph wasn't angry or resentful—he seemed to be grieving.

On suddenly hearing the news his beloved mistress had died in a car wreck, Ralph was whisked out of the home they shared (site of the many sex parties) and quickly settled into his duties at a Long Island motel. I asked who had informed him about the accident and who'd taken him to the motel. Her friends had done all this, he replied. I then inquired if he'd ever gone to her funeral, read her obituary or seen a death certificate. He'd witnessed no such thing—her friends had only claimed she was dead and had then driven him to his new location. There he was used as a cook, cleaner, houseboy, handyman and in exchange for his day's work, provided with food and shelter. I thought he must have felt isolated at the motel and asked whether he had an automobile. But Ralph didn't know how to drive, had no driver's license, and possessed no identity card which would allow him to get such a license. His lifeline was having access to the internet and learning how to search websites.

Ralph, who considered himself a slave, spent his off-work hours exploring slavery on the internet and confided he was seeking another situation. But of course, what else would a lifelong oppressed person want but freedom!

"So, Ralph, in your hopes and dreams, how do you really want to live?"

"I want to be a lady's slave," he answered calmly, with conviction.

"But why?" I was fascinated by the man.

"Because to give yourself to someone else, so entirely and fully, is the most wonderful, satisfying thing I can imagine."

I almost told him: Ralph! Go to that street in Queens where you lived. Find the house where, for over a decade, you were sequestered and not permitted to leave. Then see the dead mistress you mourn, now alive and thriving, doubtlessly wed to a fellow who doesn't want his bride to come with slave baggage!

But why should I hurt the man? Why acquaint him with cruel reality? He was possibly the purest soul I'd ever spoken to in my life. I wanted to help him, I really did—but in the end, I shirked the responsibility. As I soon learned, there wasn't just one man like Ralph living as a woman's slave in modern day America, there were many.

ELEVEN

Hardwired To Serve

WHEN I CLICKED ON AN E-MAIL FROM BRADLEY with *My Three Loves* in the subject line, three pictures appeared. The first showed me smiling demurely, wearing a pastel off-the-shoulder summer dress, my long blonde hair wind-tossed. The second displayed Bradley's overweight grown daughter, with a punk haircut and multiple tattoos, scowling while sprawled on a naugahyde sofa. The third was of his pit bull, mouth agape and drooling, wearing a thick leather collar not unlike the one I sometimes placed on his master. I thought the three photos similar to those tests of basic intelligence, where you must guess which one is out of place.

Bradley's weekdays were devoted toward making his Connecticut-based employer more money while living a comfortable suburban life as a doting grandpa. His weekends were spent with me in Manhattan shopping, dining out, taking in a play, walking around the West Village, or whatever activity I suggested. He had suddenly cut off all contact with Goddess Gina and saw Doctor Domme only sporadically, when I gave him permission. Bradley had now decided I was the mistress with whom he wanted to spend his life.

"He's a fantasy slave and not someone willing to live as a slave in real life," declared slave Clive*. Clive, a British slave I'd first begun to correspond with online, was now my frequent telephone caller and closest kinky confidant. He spoke to me almost daily (usually to disapprove of Bradley's weekend behavior) all the while instructing me how a *real* slave should comport himself. Clive claimed to be a rare "born slave," unique and pure as a unicorn, one with greater authority in all slavish matters. He called from England, where he summered—we planned to meet upon his return to the States in late August. Clive, a fifty-something retired schoolmaster, had given me his home address in nearby suburban New Jersey. Having dual U.S. and British nationality, he'd inherited his home from an aunt. "I have many relatives over there and I rather like the States, despite its deficiency of civilized behavior," he sniffed. If I called him Clive he'd correct me, as an Englishman would with the proper title to address a noble: "It's *slave* Clive."

At the same time I was discovering slavery, I was engrossed in the TV drama *Downton Abbey*. As I couldn't get enough masters and servants television, I also watched back episodes of *Upstairs, Downstairs*. In each series, the loyal house butler would often admonish a servant "not to be getting above yourself" and be mindful they were employed by their *betters*. In early twentieth century England, everyone seemed to have known their place, though social mobility soon came with social change.

But slave Clive had an arrogant air and know-it-all attitude which contrasted with his avowed self-image. "I've always believed I'm inferior to certain people who are superior, set above me in society," he confided during our first phone call.

"Oh, that's just the British class system and it's dying out. How many years have you lived over here anyway?"

"I'm retired to America a mere two years, madam." His voice was rich and plummy with perfect diction, strictly British upper-crust. It didn't surprise me to hear he'd recently ended a long teaching career—the guy seemed accustomed to being in some authority.

I disclosed to Clive how an Australian, who identified himself as a slave, had contacted me. I had asked the Aussie how he served his mistress. He replied that through a series of misfortunes, he worked as an indentured laborer in Southeast Asia and had no way out. According to the poor fellow, he toiled 18 hours a day for no pay, but had internet access once a week. The Australian was amazed to discover so many white people who actually wished to be or wanted to keep slaves.

"I told him these internet sites were for people who craved a certain kind of interpersonal scene," I confided in Clive. "He doesn't need a mistress, he needs to contact the local Australian Embassy."

"What he needs is a good attorney, madam. You must not get further along with the chap. If he's not asking you for money, it sounds like he's spending some time in an Asian jail, doubtlessly for drug dealing. Indeed, you should break off all contact."

"That never occurred to me! He says he's Australian. But because he was either in Malaysia or Indonesia—I forgot exactly where—I thought he'd been sold into slavery." Clive often displayed some wisdom or worldly sophistication.

"A nonconsensual slave is not a true slave, not in my mind, as they have been coerced by various means. They are, in effect, abducted prisoners forced to work against their will—and for absolutely nothing, on pain of death or disability. Indeed, why should they not speak out?" He was typically so eloquent and theatrical, I could imagine slave Clive having a career on the London stage, or in the British Parliament.

"What you need, madam, is a *consensual* slave. Someone to look after you and your interests. He would shop for your daily needs, cook your meals, clean your house, draw your bath, massage your weary body."

"But I already have slave Bradley plus a cleaning lady." I had already informed Clive that Bradley lived north of New York but spent weekends with me in Manhattan.

"*Slave* Bradley. I don't suppose he sleeps with you, does he?"

"Oh, no, but sometimes, when he spends the night, he sleeps in the living room all by himself."

"And he's not a pussy pumper?" inquired an indignant Clive.

"No, Bradley would never want something like insertion. He's a true submissive man. But there's no need for a full-time slave here. I don't do much cooking with all the good prepared foods and take-out we have in Manhattan. Besides, a lot of these slaves I find online experience slavery as a fetish. They're just kinksters."

"*Kinksters*, madam?" he repeated, as if offended. "I am offering you a rather serious proposal which has no relation with perversion whatsoever but everything to do with service, loyalty, dedication and obedience. Some people, like myself, are born to serve others. Our happiness is derived from making a major difference in the lives of our owners. I am seeking, madam, to become whole at last, to finally live my birthright vocation. Being a Southern gentlewoman, you understand how slavery does not have to be a force for evil." My Southern accent was still strong, even after living in New York for 40 years.

Clive continued in his melodious manner of speaking. "The best slaves are not those who've been abducted and sold but who are naturally, genetically predisposed to a life of slavery. People like myself, well, we're like homosexuals and others born a certain way. There's just no changing us. I have long ago accepted what I am. Now that I'm retired, I need a dominant female who can handle the benevolent ownership of one born as an inferior submissive entity."

"I realize it's difficult to find a woman slave owner and I've noticed many guys online looking for one. Have you tried dating a really demanding, bossy lady or a control freak?"

"Slaves don't *date*, madam," he replied in a cutting fashion. "Some like myself are rather damaged through exposure to the polluting influence of freedom, which depletes our natural submission. I would devote myself to enhancing the life of a deserving owner and make her life more rewarding, free of domestic drudgery. Why should my superiors be demeaned by performing mindless tasks when they could be engaged in more fruitful activities? Now, can't you see yourself owning a slave like me?"

"Honestly, slave Bradley does anything I tell him to do when helping around the house. He kneels, lowers his eyes and kisses my feet when he enters. He walks behind me in public and goes ahead of me only to open doors. He takes me out to the restaurants I choose and brings home my favorite wine. So, I'd say I'm all set in the slave department."

"Don't be ridiculous calling that man a *slave*," Clive spat. "Didn't you say he lived with you only on weekends, worked at a job in Connecticut, and is also used by another domme?"

"Yes, I want him to hold down a responsible position and he has one. Bradley occasionally helps this sickly, infirm pro-domme, but he always asks my permission first for the loan-out."

"You must understand, madam, a slave cannot see who it pleases, say what it pleases, or come and go as it pleases," Clive continued in a crisp tone." A slave is *property* belonging to its owner; as such he is only entitled to basic needs. A slave runs your home but does not become a part of your social life."

Though I found slave Clive fascinating, I would not further accept his phone calls until we'd first had a video chat. As his computer didn't have this capability, he agreed to visit a local internet cafe which did, finally allowing us to see one another. "Good morning to you, madam," he began with his usual confidence. "Now I appreciate the fact you're rather new to the situation, but you must understand *millions* do this. No one should enter such an arrangement unless secure in the knowledge this lifestyle suits their character and they'd benefit from it immensely." A male appeared on my computer screen who spoke in the inimitable way I'd heard for the past few weeks. Finally I could see slave Clive—this fellow with the receding hairline. He wore a conservative white dress shirt open at the neck, as if he'd decided to leave off the necktie for an interview. Though the video image was somewhat distorted, he had pleasant features and looked entirely normal.

"Yes, but I imagine you can adapt and learn to compromise," I replied.

"Not about that which feeds and strengthens a slave's purpose. Things like direction, discipline and service. About these there can be no compromise, madam, because when they are lacking, slavery itself cannot long be sustained." He spoke with a stirring locution which could have come straight from the pulpit. "You are an attractive woman indeed. It is only natural vanilla or dominant men will pretend to be submissive in order to get their cocks into your pussy and claim you as yet another conquest."

"Watch your tongue with that language!" I told his computer image. "Your assumption is entirely untrue—I entertain slaves and submissive men only!"

"I imagine most of these so-called slaves are merely submissives. You see, madam, the BDSM community has hijacked slavery and now the word *slave* has lost its true meaning. Real owners do not parade their slaves about conferences or dungeons alongside members of the leather community and such. Ownership is a private, not public, matter."

"So you're saying these slaves exist in a sort of shadow society?"

"Let's just say one of the differences between submissives and slaves is there's no sane, safe and consensual activity guidelines in slavery. Slavery is not *play*. There are no *sessions* in slavery. Slavery, madam, is like submission but times one hundred," he emphasized with a certain solemnity. "I see you have much to learn. In the meanwhile, make sure your submissive gentleman worships you with due humility," intoned Clive before terminating our video connection.

Clive's severe style of slavery was not what I wanted with Bradley. We spent the next Sunday morning viewing bucolic country homes featured by realtors online. "*Aw-w*, look at this old stone house with a well out back," he enthused. "It's on an acre and a half and so well tended." I stuck my forefinger under his leather collar and gave it a tug towards me. With this nasty little choking action, Bradley moaned in pleasure. But when I let go of his collar, his interest returned to my laptop. "Who wouldn't want to live there?"

A Manhattan resident who loves big cities, I thought to myself as he clicked on the next prospective dwelling.

"What you and I need is more space," Bradley declared. I liked the space we already had—an hour and a half travel time between our two homes.

"Do you collar him?" Clive pried when he called on Monday.

"At the beginning of the weekend, I usually place his collar on after he first enters, when he's kneeling. But he doesn't wear it outside."

"And why not?"

"I don't want strangers noticing it. He walks a bit behind me on the street but I don't want him on display looking like a kinkster."

"You should always walk about with your head held high and your bosom out, proud you have a slave! Believe me, you will certainly not be alone as a slave owner in New York. And do you know *why* a slave is collared? It is ancient custom and tradition, madam. It shows the slave is owned property when the slave is not naked and shackled. A collar identifies the slave and also who owns it. The device is normally welded or locked upon the neck."

"No, Bradley is a slave *lite*. He wears a leather dog collar I got on eBay and it's got this rhinestone heart on it."

"Disgusting." I could sense his shudder even over the Atlantic Ocean. "One is most certainly not to imply any loving feelings towards their slave! A slave is to be thought of, spoken to and treated as such at all times. Its submission and obedience are demonstrated by adopting servile postures. Remember this well, madam: Female supremacy is all about absolute power and control over men and using them for whatever purpose a woman may want."

"Really? I thought that was marriage."

"Actually, you should marry your submissive fellow, move to the country with him, live in a big house—and then I could be the slave of a couple!" he merrily suggested.

"You've got to be kidding!"

"Not in the least. He has some money and he does as he's told—at least on weekends. You can feel safe with gentleman B. as he can give you added financial security. He'd be a fine husband for you, just as I'd be an excellent slave beast for you both. Of course, I'd contribute towards the joint living arrangement. A modern day slave pulls its own weight and is never a drain on the household's financial resources. A slave should buy its own health, car and life insurance plus pay towards its room, board and utility bills. Keep in mind a slave never interferes and always stays in the background."

"But I like things as they are with Bradley—living in our separate homes and seeing each other on weekends. We have our little rituals. He comes to my place, we have some wine, he takes me out. After dinner he draws my bath, sometimes he bathes me..."

Clive interrupted. "And does he don the slave's hood, madam?"

"No, he dresses conservatively. I've never seen him wear a hoodie."

"Traditionally, when bathing their mistress, slaves wore hoods without any fabric cut out for the eyes, so they could never see their naked betters. That is the method I have adopted. I also recommend having many lit and flickering candles about the bath."

"Candles are forbidden. Remember, I've got two cats and they jump about like grasshoppers, so it's just too dangerous. My cats rule the roost, their safety comes first and you'd have to feel the same."

"As you prefer, madam."

"So, you'll do as you're instructed? Good! Are you a cat person?"

"That is not a problem, madam. I rather like cats and have had extensive experience with them. Now, if ownership is something you wish to pursue, because it is most suitable for your psyche and natural dominance, it's important you go ahead with it. After all, we can't change ourselves."

He was right about not being able to change, at least in my case. A serial-dating spinster with four decades of boyfriends behind me, I was becoming bored by Bradley, who was forever telling me, with a multitude of it's-not-abouts, what it was like to be a slave. "It's not about how you look, it's about how you care," he'd mutter as we hunted for his perfect jacket. Ever since I'd insisted on his wardrobe makeover, shopping for men's clothes had taken up a good part of our weekend's leisure time. I'd taught him to avoid synthetics in favor of natural fibers like cotton, wool and silks. I'd gotten him into wine and interested in traveling overseas. "I do love being taught and influenced by you," he confessed as we stopped for some sorbet. "It adds so much to our mistress-slave dynamic. Because slavery is not about contempt, slavery is about respect."

I wondered whether he really did respect me, as he was forever yapping about successful women—not successful men—in a specific reverent way, one almost fetishistic. Claiming he was done with Goddess Gina, sometime he'd beg my permission to see Doctor Domme, terming it a loan-out and emphasizing I was his owner. (In reality, ownership is a lengthy process with a written contract and rigid rules, nothing like the casual arrangement I had with Bradley.) He specifically asked to spend one Sunday later in the month cleaning for her.

"Sure you can. You'd feel really bad if Doctor Domme died suddenly and you hadn't been responsive to her. Just don't tell her my name and where I live. I've been there and done that with guys' old girlfriends—they're almost as bad as male stalkers!"

"Oh, she would never do such a thing. It's not about her being so into me; she just enjoys having me around. I can't figure her out. I don't know whether it's her illness or because she's been a pro-domme for so long—but something has made her lose her humanity. Maybe if we spent some time together looking through her high school yearbook or saw pictures from her youth, this could bring out her hard-to-handle, deep emotions. I'm not ashamed to shed a man tear every once in a while, so maybe such a stimulus will prompt the release she needs. Because slavery is not about denying yourself, slavery is about being open."

Slave Clive also lectured me on what it meant to be a slave. "A free man has certain rights no inferior submissive nonentity should ever have!"

Over 40 years earlier, while attending college in Georgia, I'd heard a few frat boys rail against racial integration, groaning they'd like to "send them back to Africa" or how Blacks were best suited to be slaves. But Clive insisted he "wanted and needed traditional slavery as it was once practiced in the Southern states." He not only loved the fact I was Southern by birth and breeding, he professed to admire the antebellum system of plantation slavery. "As an authentic Southern gentlewoman, surely you must understand the age-old need for slavery." He always pronounced *slavery* fully drawn out, each syllable distinctly pronounced with a certain sense of grandeur, as some of his countrymen would have said the word *royalty* in decades past. "And consensual slavery is still being practiced in the South."

"Come on, there aren't any Blacks in America who are currently involved in slavery!" I erupted in giggles as slave Clive seldom failed to amuse me.

"It is no laughing matter, madam. They call themselves The House of Blue Flames and if you don't believe me, I will send you the contact information for their tribe. But you must first get your own house in order. About Mr. B: Always make him be naked indoors in your presence! Get him to prepare all your meals! Insist he adopt servile postures like kneeling, bowing his head, kissing your feet! Have him avoid direct eye contact with you! Demand he perform cunnilingus on you! Tell him he now belongs to you alone, he is your property and you *own* him! And make him do demeaning chores, even if they don't need to be done."

"What's a demeaning chore as opposed to housework?"

"You've some cats, you say, and I suppose they shit and piss. Well, use your imagination! Simply treat him mean to keep him keen—but in a subtle, sensual and feminine manner," he advised in his most mellifluous voice.

A few hours later, Clive sent me contact information for The House of Blue Flames and I visited their website. As he had described, they appeared to be a Black group who practiced slavery in South Carolina. I read online how their slaves must give "absolute submission to Master of the House" and their master has "absolute authority over the slaves of his House." They'd been operating for over a decade, with Master Sable having acquired slave dreamy, slave meira, slave butterfly and one or two others. As a bunch of Blacks owning Black slaves, they were not alone, claiming they were "in harmonious alliance with several other Houses we loosely refer to as Our Family," all located in the South.

I had to hand it to Clive, he usually knew what he was talking about. And bizarre as it may seem, his information generally proved reality-based. Compared to many other kinksters I'd met online, slave Clive was both experienced and rational. "When you return to America next month, let's have lunch," I suggested. "You live fairly close to where I work during the day."

"You do not take a mere slave to lunch with you, madam. A slave is *property*, not a friend to socialize with."

"But I like going out to eat and sharing a bottle of wine with Bradley. You're just so rigid. Maybe it's from all those years you taught school. How do you adjust, going from schoolteacher to slave?"

"We often begin our lives engaged in things other than the purpose for which we were born. This gives us life experience before we commence our respective birthright vocation."

"You're overqualified and way too educated for slavery."

"Not so. But I have many skills which can be utilized in my owner's service, all to make her life more fulfilled. And with a slave like me, you can let loose your dark side in private," he offered in a lower tone.

"I don't really have a dark side."

"Oh, pish posh! You, madam, were actually born to live with and own a naked, collared and chained slave beast—and if you don't believe me, examine your thoughts on female dominance and inferior male servitude. Males have this lowly place in your life as mere objects to serve, worship, obey and suffer for you! Why then did you learn to utilize punishment techniques if not to cause pain and maintain control?"

I could hardly tell him I began investigating femdom as part of my job. The *Leg Action* editor before me had never been to Paddles and didn't even know where the club was. No one at work told me when writing for the magazine, I had to practice what I preached. Clive was right—I had a natural predilection for dominating men. But he had to know I was both cautious and selective. "Ladies never make future behavior promises with guys they haven't met—not unless they're those fat women who correspond with prisoners. And that's just not me!"

"So the answer is *no*, madam?"

"I already have slave Bradley."

"That one is only a make-believe slave, not a true slave! Honestly, do you want a prissy, sissy weekend slave—or one like me, who would care for you, speak up on your behalf and look after your interests? I think we should discuss some pre-ownership agreement parameters, madam."

The arrangement did not sound unappealing. "O.K., just what would this entail?"

"Although you are getting much guidance from me, madam, you must tailor ownership to your own needs and personality. You see, there are many different slavery philosophies such as Gorean, Gothic, and Old Guard. But rest assured, I would never bring you into disrepute or betray my owner's business to anyone. Nor would I utter any word or do any deed which could possibly ridicule my owner. I will be a credit to you, madam, and do nothing detrimental to you or your wellbeing. And I would willingly sign a confidentiality agreement."

"It just sounds too permanent for me, even worse than marriage."

"The fact is, madam, this is far better, as you can look before you leap. The first day of meeting there is a physical inspection, then a period of engaging in background and health checks. There can be a trial period of one week to one month, as you wish. Next comes a probationary period of three months to one year—and all that comes before permanent ownership."

"Oh, I see. There is some trying out and an adjustment period."

"Quite so, madam. Suffice it to say owning a real slave, and not a weekend let's pretend slave, will change your life for the better—if it's high quality and knows its place."

As he spoke, a pleasant sensation overcame me. Why not be an owner? I wouldn't be just an ordinary middle-class senior citizen. I would be a woman who had her every need catered to, and every wish obeyed. The opening bars to the *Downton Abbey* theme song trilled in my head.

TWELVE

Who's The Slave Here?

ONE EARLY MONDAY EVENING, I RECEIVED A CALL from slave Clive, who'd tried to reach me the day before. He asked where I'd been.

"Oh, I was at the movies with Bradley. Why didn't you leave me a message?"

"Movie theaters! Well, I imagined as much. Engaged in your fantasy role play scenario with Mr. B. Why should I interrupt? I trust you had a pleasant time," he inquired in his snotty way.

Bradley and I had planned to see an early evening movie. We arrived at the multiplex, bought tickets for the show and walked in to a film already well in progress. As it ended about 45 minutes after we were seated, we stayed to see the beginning. But as the theater's policy required everyone to file out, management targeted the two of us. Although I'd gotten the movie time for Thursday, not the weekend, I railed about how we'd been sold tickets for a screening halfway over and insisted they give us some freebies to acknowledge their mistake. The theater manager handed ten free passes to Bradley, who had said nothing throughout the confrontation. "Mistress, the way you handled that guy—you were magnificent!" Bradley had enthused afterward, handing me five of these tickets and keeping an equal number for himself.

Clive crisply summed up the Bradley situation: "The chap takes you out and about, when he should actually *pay* for the time he spends with you, this part-time slave. A *real* slave expects his lady owner to benefit from his slavery, both emotionally and financially, by paying part room and board. Trotting about town with a real slave is just not done, madam. It is not your lover, friend or acquaintance but owned *property* and should be treated accordingly."

"But just last week you were advising me to marry Bradley," I reminded him.

"Indeed. He'd be your husband and I would be your slave. And there can be no sex between an owner and her slave."

"What about all the cunnilingus you're always talking about? What's that?"

"If a slave is performing cunnilingus to pleasure its owner, it's a *service* and not sex, as such. Know this, madam—no real slave is or should be a sex slave. Having sex with a slave is far, far worse than pedophilia, as it is bestiality. You can use a free person or, in rare instances, a submissive man for purposes of copulation; but a slave can only give cunnilingus or massage, perhaps suckle the breasts if you order it to do so."

"Then all those pictures you sent me of dicks enclosed in plastic and metal, the chastity devises—I know it's a major fetish among submissive men, but what has it to do with slavery?"

"You are a mature, intelligent and refined lady. Why then, do you not comprehend these are genital restraints? Their purpose is to permanently deny erection so the slave can concentrate on its servile labor. You should place your friend, Mr. B., in strict chastity to ensure he does not stray and only *you* have access to what would become your very own masculine genitals. There should be no argument over the matter of locking him up, madam. It ensures loyalty and service to only one woman."

"My Mr. B. channels his sexuality into housework," I explained. "Since I have a regular cleaning lady, he cheats on me by cleaning another domme's dirty apartment. That's fine by me—the sound of a vacuum cleaner drives me to distraction. But Bradley is so happy cleaning, he's sort of sexualized a certain apron he wears. He's a basic service bottom and his penis isn't even an issue."

"If I may be so bold to say—I think you may be deluding yourself, madam."

"You're right, the penis is *always* the issue. I wouldn't even know what to do with a chastity thing, they look kind of complicated."

"Don't be ridiculous. Securing already assembled chastity restraints is hardly difficult. You are making much over absolutely nothing. The question is this: How will you feel when the time comes to place a made-to-measure chastity restraint on a set of male genitalia and lock the device in place?"

"I suppose you're saying you have such a thing, slave Clive. You *do* have one, right?"

"One? No, madam. I own five."

That weekend Bradley dressed me for dinner. I raised my arms so he could lower the silk shift over my head, settle it about my hips and zip up the back. I then brought up the matter of his chastity, and continued to speak on the subject while he sat on my dressing stool. I placed one foot, then the other, in his lap. As he fastened the buckles of my high heeled sandals, I watched his expression change from bliss to panic. Reality had just caught up to fantasy. As expected, Bradley claimed he'd love to "lock it away" for me—but as he lived an hour and a half from Manhattan, he could only wear the device during our weekends together. Bradley, a hyper-groomed health nut, was well aware how putting his genitals behind metal or plastic for days at a time—with no key holder in sight—would be unhygienic. I thought weekend chastity was as weak as weekend submission, and knew I had no real control over this man.

"Perfectly understandable," slave Clive acknowledged. "I see Gentleman B. is no fool, realizing one must have access to a key holder for bathing and other practical purposes. Now tell me, you *do* practice CBT on your submissive boyfriend, don't you?" His tone was both dangerous and seductive, a tiger's purr.

"Yes, the most severe kind."

"Ah, tell me how."

"Well, I totally ignore his penis and pretend it isn't even there. As a result, he claims to always suffer this sexual frustration—though he seems to enjoy it."

"You would not get away with such nonsense as a slave owner, madam. Cock and ball torture is vital in maintaining the control dynamic, ensuring the slave both knows and keeps its place. Even the best slave will have times when it slips. You do CBT then—that's how to get those standards tip-top again. And it will keep the slave focused. I say now, perhaps one day you could host a Cock and Balls Torture Ladies Supper. Now, you had some women over for bridge last week..."

"Reality, slave Clive! Reality!" I barked, interrupting him. "Didn't you claim you'd do nothing to bring me into disrepute?"

"My conduct and deportment must be of a high order when your friends visit. Indeed, madam, you must seem to be very much in charge."

"But they're not dommes! Now let's see if you can wrap your brain around your own physical welfare. Don't you know there are areas down there that should never be hit?"

"Oh, don't go on about the safety malarkey. The entire penis and testicles can be disciplined without causing injury if they're in the flaccid state. Despite its fragile appearance, the entire lot is fairly resilient."

"And what makes you even think my friends would enjoy torturing a penis?"

"Because most heterosexual vanilla women respond well to the eye candy of a muscular male body in a locked chastity restraint, wearing a metal collar and in shackles. You imagine it may shock them—but some would rather enjoy having me cook them dinner and serve it in an obedient, attentive manner. It's perfectly natural for a slave to perform the functions of a servant and be protective of its owner. There is nothing bizarre about it, not in the least. I'd like your lady guests to think—indeed, I too, must acquire a slave to enhance my life."

"Look, I'm not suggesting you be kept closeted. In the future, I intend to be open about my lifestyle. But I know what most women will accept. About those pictures I received of you in leather outfits—well, any Manhattan woman would think you're a gay guy off to the Crisco Disco. Eye candy here is not leather, it's GQ. That's a men's fashion magazine, for your information. The near-naked, muscular male form is something they can see any day at the gym, and will not impress my friends as would a nice clothed appearance."

"Oh dear, what prudish women they are. They must be such a frigid lot, I pity their husbands."

"And what's this about shackles? Aren't those worn on the legs? I'm not having you dragging chains about, scratching up my nice wood floors! How do you possibly imagine women would like seeing such a bizarre thing?"

"I think most women would enjoy it as a bit of light-hearted, healthy fun."

"Oh yeah? I think they'd run for the hills. And what's healthy about torturing a penis or testicles?"

He cleared his throat, as if readying the most persuasive point in an oratory. "It's proven to be rather good exercise for slave genitals, in ways other than sexual stimulus."

There was the matter of the penis lead, which he claimed was the only practical way to walk a slave. "The neck is a rather delicate part of the body and too much jerking can damage it. It is more comfortable for the male if the mistress secures her slave's center parts to lead him about. A penis lead lies lower on the spine than a collar, it's easier to handle and the genitals are never harmed by it."

Slave Clive had an excuse for every kinky behavior—a rationale couched in terms of proper master-slave decorum or in the interest of one's health. "I would like for you to take a leap forward, put aside your distaste for what you call sadism and practice some Therapeutic Flogging. Most dominant women who try it actually enjoy it, and are hooked, despite an initial reluctance."

"Therapeutic Flogging. Shouldn't the mistress choose her own style of chastisement?"

"Indeed, madam. It is a matter of trial and error plus personal preference. But I subscribe to the quadrant method because it is more sensible."

"And how is this more sensible?" I loved to challenge him, yet he usually mistook my sordid curiosity as genuine interest.

"Because it delivers an equal distribution of lash strokes. Here's how: You use lipstick or a felt tip pen to draw 24 quadrants on the male servile anatomy. There's four each to the right and left upper back, four to the right and left buttock, and four more to both the left and right rear thigh. A total of 24 with the 25th to the male genitalia. You must use some analgesic spray before starting. Post punishment, apply an ice cold towel every 15 or 30 minutes to all the quadrant areas. This cools down any heat from the lash strokes and you avoid bruising this way. You see? It's simple!"

"No, it sounds like a lot of effort for God knows what purpose."

"The purpose of executing such a flogging, madam, is to enhance the general wellbeing of the owner. The actual power a lady has to inflict various levels of pain, while witnessing her slave suffer—this can trigger intense erotic responses in the owner. A three-dimensional tranquility is created which results in an intense sexual fulfillment. And for this to be achieved, the slave creature must endure prolonged pain as a sacrifice for his owner's benefit." He spoke with the fervor of a true believer.

"So what does the slave get out of it?"

"There is, madam, a release of certain stressful anxieties, resulting from the production of endorphins. These are very positive health-enhancing chemicals which give a feeling of energy in the slave body. They also reduce the sensation of pain."

He was describing how masochism actually works, with the sufferer desirous of their endorphin-based high as if it were a drug—though it is doubtful increased pain is required to trigger the desired level of euphoria (as in a drug addiction). I began to realize why many hardwired masochists speak of their kink in terms of wellness.

One of Clive's main sources for health and fitness information was Other World Kingdom (usually referred to as OWK), a BDSM resort located on the outskirts of Prague. In the way I would tell friends, "I learned about taking Senna for constipation at Johns Hopkins," dropping the name of the world-renowned hospital where I'd had surgery, slave Clive would declare with like pride: "That's the way they did it at OWK."

Now only an internet site, during the years between 1997 to 2008, OWK operated as a Disneyland for dommes. Actually a grand estate, the castle complex featured a Queen's Palace with banquet hall, library, throne room, gym, basement prison, and torture chambers. Well-tended grounds and outdoor facilities provided horses, stables and an indoor riding ring. Additional amenities included a restaurant, pub, nightclub, guest rooms, swimming pool and more torture chambers. OWK was the residence of its absolute monarch, Queen Patricia I, and operated as a sovereign matriarchy. Under Queen Patricia, Lady Citizens ruled with absolute authority, displaying cruelty and contempt as many (not all) men were reduced to sniveling, groveling lesser beings.

OWK was never a part of the Czech Republic, which bordered it, but a micronation unrecognized by other world governments—like a much smaller kinkster North Korea. What separates a micronation from a mere imaginary country is some claim of rule over a physical territory, which was OWK's seven plus acres. Some micronations have their own currency as did OWK (called the DOM), their own flag (OWK's flag had the biological symbol for female front and center), and their own coat of arms (OWK's included the motto Women Over Men). Then there was the stirring, fully orchestrated OWK national anthem, a fitting score for an IMAX film centering on a medieval castle plus a dragon or two.

Primary among OWK's many rules was how one must never look directly at the Queen. People there would sometimes sense her presence, especially when she was carried about the grounds on a palanquin held aloft by several slave men. Worshipped as the ultimate symbol of female superiority, few realized their Queen was merely a woman married to the dominant man who owned this femdom theme park. The OWK government had a Treasury, Queen's Court, Queen's Guard and many sundry funky functions.

Just a step below the queen were the Lady Citizens, regarded as nobility. To become an OWK citizen, a woman had to obey the many

OWK rules and regulations, spend at least five nights in the area of the Queen's Palace (always a pricey proposition), and own at least one male slave. Ownership was initially taken seriously; OWK used to keep a formal slave register. (Although in its later years, a man could get on the OWK slave register simply by ordering BDSM gear from their website.)

As for the males of the realm, they were regarded as either Queen's Subjects or of the lower class, a slave. Queens's Subjects followed OWK law, obeyed the Queen, paid taxes, and had many rights. These included the freedom to travel, own property, have children, and state opinions. By comparison, the male slaves had forfeited all rights, becoming property of either the Queen or one of the Lady Citizens, and were viewed as being on the level of a farm animal. It was exactly the way these slave guys liked it.

Just as vacationers can customize an adventure trek to their own activity level, one could tailor the OWK experience. Some men reported a fun weekend of BDSM games and contests. (These included voting on which sub had the most impressive marks and bruises on his ass, or participating in the popular Slave Olympics.) Others remembered a more traumatic weekend of containment in small locked cages, being physically restrained while receiving countless severe blows and deprived of food. The most challenging (and therefore expensive) OWK experience was typically paid for by a dominant woman and tailored to make her man maximally submissive. This programming lasted for several weeks and utilized many more of the pro-dommes who lived and worked there. Through much custom-made degradation coupled with a series of ultra-sadistic measures, the deluxe OWK treatment was guaranteed to break even the toughest submissive male, reducing him to a mindless creature who only served, obeyed and suffered at the hands of dominant females. If a woman wanted to turn her sub into a slave, she only had to throw a few thousand dollars at OWK and lure the guy to Eastern Europe for a quaint countryside vacation.

Housing many prosperous men, even some captains of commerce, OWK included kinksters (both dommes and subs alike) from several staid, civilized European countries and other nations worldwide. Slave

Clive had joined them on occasion. He spoke of OWK with the appreciative nostalgia of a grown man remembering the final bonfire at summer camp, when he had bidden his little bunkmates goodbye. He earnestly recalled the human horse rides at OWK and suggested we engage in the same. "Riding the slave beast on a saddle backpack or attaching it to a buggy are worthwhile leisure pursuits. Being outdoors, in the fresh air, on the back of a strong naked slave who has stamina would benefit you, madam, both physically and emotionally."

I'd seen some OWK horseplay pictures showing men drawing carts in place of horses. And plenty of OWK males wearing masks more grotesque than those of Mexican Lucha Libre wrestlers. Others had been placed on a wooden wheel of pain, with clothespins attached to their nipples and scrotums. More were chained to a pillory while a lit candle licked at their genitals—or used as human furniture with a mistress atop him, her spike heel resting upon his face. For slave Clive, it was all an ass-kissing, boot-licking, balls-kicking good time. OWK was his Club Med.

According to Clive, Bradley would benefit from an OWK stay, but the complex had been recently shut down and offered for sale. "People don't realize certain males must simply be taken off the streets to be whipped, stripped, shackled and put to use as the slave beasts of dominant females. If you ask me, mothers are to blame for not training their submissive sons in the art of obedience to women," slave Clive opined.

Bradley had never been to Other World Kingdom, although he had traveled within Europe. The following weekend Bradley went online to show me more prospective homes, these now located much further from New York City. "It's where you can get more house for the money," he muttered. We both realized what he claimed to want (be my slave and have me dominate him 24/7) was at odds with his current living situation. I had never been to his house. After we'd been dating for about two months, his scary-looking grown daughter moved in, residing there alongside the scary dog. He showed me two places which interested him: a four bedroom on a cul-de-sac and a six bedroom in the countryside.

Bradley initially told me the daughter had two young sons (aged two and four) and worked in fashion. The boys lived with her ex-husband, their father, with whom she was actively engaged in a child custody battle. Sometimes Bradley would fume about those irrational accusations the ex-husband had made about his daughter's fitness to be a mother. Of course, it was Bradley who paid her many legal bills. As I later learned, the daughter didn't actually work in the fashion industry but as a suburban retail store clerk. "She's a wonderful mother," Bradley claimed pridefully, as we had our Sunday morning coffee. "And very fertile."

"You've poured lots of money into her custody case. Think she'll win?"

"As it is now, she has only visitation rights, not even joint custody. It's worth the money I've spent just to contest those outrageous charges made against her. So I wouldn't be at all surprised if we get custody."

We? "And what will you do then?"

"Then I guess it's the big country house with the pond out back. That's why I'm waiting to buy. Things must be settled in court before I know how much room we need."

"I thought you wanted to be a lady's slave—but now I see you're mainly a grandfather!"

"Mistress, I am willing to serve you always and am completely yours in my slave heart and soul. But I must defer my living preferences to those who can give life. This doesn't mean I don't want you there with us. You can still be my mistress, boss me around, and all the while have a great family living experience."

"You know how kids irritate me!" I spat. "I may find them annoying but at least I admit it. And I'd never allow my cats to be around toddlers, who can be so mindlessly cruel to small animals, much less a big dog, one that's part pit bull."

"But we'd be in a huge house with spacious grounds. And I'd offer you a 60/40 arrangement."

I had to ask Bradley what this was, thinking perhaps 60/40 was some hedge fund term. With most guys I'd recently known, it probably meant I'd torture over half of his penis, leaving the rest unharmed. "I'd contribute the most towards our living expenses. My 60 to your 40, Mistress," he replied.

"And what would your daughter put in if she's living there with her kids?"

"Come on, you don't expect a young mother, making minimum wage and saddled with young children, to be on equal footing, do you?"

"This 40 percent expected from me—does my percentage go for the home's mortgage, property taxes and house repairs?"

"Of course. Plus there's gas, water and electricity..."

I cut him off before he could continue. "And the title of this house you're seeking to buy—the property would be in whose name?"

"I'm making the down payment so it would be in my name and in the name of my daughter. She has such bad credit, she can't buy any property on her own. But hey, you'd still be mistress of the house and I'd be your slave. Because slavery isn't about being unable to escape—slavery is about being committed."

"Look, anyone who's worked hard, in order to live in Manhattan, would be reluctant to leave for a lesser situation."

"Do you think being around nature and fresh air, loved ones and a family is worse than living alone? Kids are great—they have a certain energy."

"I don't live alone. I live with my loved ones, my cats. Little kids make me nervous. As for energy, I live in Manhattan, where I'll always stay." I actually preferred being solely in the company of my cats, which was what others called alone.

Slave Clive owned a five bedroom house in a New Jersey suburb just outside New York. It was also conveniently near where I worked. When I requested the address, he hadn't hesitated and noted: "It's nicely set back from the street and surrounded by lots of shrubbery, so privacy isn't an issue." When I entered the address into Google Earth, a corner lot house appeared. So this is slave Clive's lair, I thought, while spying the property he'd inherited. Large but plain, it certainly looked as if someone's aunt had lived there. "We can live together as mistress and slave in Manhattan. On some weekends, my house can also be your house. I could install a jacuzzi for my owner."

It was all fantasy, of course. We'd never even met. But the arrangement he spoke of sounded more promising than the situation Bradley offered. Although slave Clive's proposition included a trial period, I wondered whether I could handle living with such an intense fellow on a daily basis, or if I was even cut out to be an owner.

He had informed me a workshop on master/slave interaction would be held in lower Manhattan the very next month. I agreed to register, learn what I could, and perhaps get some much needed advice. "Just so we're on the same page," I told Clive.

"If you wish to own and rule over a slave, to use and abuse that slave, treat it as a slave should be treated—then yes, madam, we are most certainly on the same page. "Women rule and men obey. Surely it has always been the way."

If only.

THIRTEEN

The Real Slaves Of New York

WHY HAD I RECEIVED AN E-MAIL FROM A GROUP called the Master/slave Development Center? I'd temporarily forgotten how, just a few weeks prior, I'd registered and pre-paid for their workshop entitled "Power, Authority, Leadership and Management in M/s Relationships."

Bradley had been encouraging about my decision to attend a workshop for slave owners. Slave Clive seemed enthusiastic. "You'll tell them a true slave, a *born slave*, is coming over from England for your inspection and to begin a trial period, won't you?"

"Right, I won't forget to tell them you are a born slave—how since your early boyhood, you've never felt you were anything other than a slave, which is your birthright vocation."

The workshop was held in a large Tribeca loft with kitchen facilities plus a lounge containing sofas, tables, and Aeron chairs. There was a podium and microphone for speakers. The attendees appeared as a cross section of average citizens, not looking or dressing as Paddles regulars or those who had attended TES-Fest. Only one person, a woman, wore leather. With eighteen registrants, only four were women; of those four, three (including me) appeared to be over fifty years old. Although I'd told Clive there would be no slaves there, three female slaves busied themselves in the kitchen preparing coffee and tea, plus breakfast bagels and croissants.

My name tag, printed with my scene name, was handed to me by the group's leader, Sir Stephen, who was seated at a front table. "Mistress Pussycat," he read, now looking up as if appraising me. "It's a pleasure to have you here. Now please try out these chairs. I've had two brought in especially for you, so see which you prefer."

I'd forgotten how I had written him about my sitting disability, explaining I'd had my tailbone amputated and could only sit on soft chairs. "Sir Stephen, how considerate of you." A tall, good looking man in his early sixties, he was unconventionally dressed. His high cut pants had no belt, but were held by a pair of suspenders with a Y-shaped elastic piece in back. A black cravat parted the neck of his collarless shirt and a gold watch fob visibly snaked from his vest pocket. I imagined he'd left the frock coat at home.

I'd say his style was Steampunk if he had been 30 or 40 years younger and had a hipster sense of irony. But there was none of that with the straightforward Sir Stephen, just reverence for a bygone era and way of life. He ruled a strict Victorian household alongside his slave of 13 years, slave Marianne*, who I'd noticed taking charge of the conference room kitchen. Short and round, her dumpling face cheerful and smiling, she wore a black pinafore with a white Peter Pan collar at the neck and a starched white apron. The woman came across not as homely but more as homespun, and seemed more than content, just genuinely happy to be of service.

In the conference literature, Sir Stephen was described as a master and a "het," as were the other males in the group. There are so many gay men in master-slave relationships, especially in the New York City area, heterosexual males found it necessary to identify themselves as *hets*. The M/s Development Center was but one of three local groups dedicated to consensual slavery. There was MAsT: Metro New York (for heterosexuals) and its offshoot chapter, MAsT NYC (for homosexuals), both fully functioning with sizable memberships, meetings, scheduled activities and elected officers. (MAsT is the acronym for Masters

And slaves Together.) In addition, DomSubFriends had both gay and straight slaves with their masters alongside a lively, involved group of non-owner dominants and submissives.

Sir Stephen had been a founding member of MAsT: Metro New York, just one of 70 MAsT chapters in America. (There are also seven MAsT chapters outside the United States, with a presence in Canada and Australia.) Inside a three-ring notebook, I found Sir Stephen's *curriculum vitae*, along with the credentials of other workshop lecturers. His lifestyle awards and affiliations were many, but among the highlights were these nuggets: "He was honored to be the recipient of the title International Master 2005 and Northeast Master 2004" and "he was nominated in 2006, 2007, 2008, 2009 and 2010 in various categories for the Pantheon of Leather Awards." (I knew these folks took their master-slave business seriously, but had no idea there were awards given.)

Sir Stephen was currently devoting much of his time to this Master/slave Development Center, where he was a founding member. As I perused the well-organized course material, I imagined an MBA degree must be somewhere in Sir Stephen's background.

In his opening remarks, Sir Stephen acknowledged everyone needed training and recognition but this workshop was for masters, not slaves. Even the word *master*, he noted, grew out of the medieval guild system. Boys who went into a guild were taught a skill. If and when they produced a worthy piece, it was judged and pronounced to be a masterpiece, its maker becoming a master. With a nod to political correctness, he noted *master* would be used in this workshop, though it also pertained to dominant females who used the title Lady or Mistress. He further explained how there were subsets of consensual slavery. One, for instance, was the Daddy/boy relationship so popular among gay men. There was also, for those bottoms who did not identify with being human, the trainer/pet arrangement.

Master Peter*, a former career military officer with 15 years behind him in the lifestyle, conducted the workshop on Power. Like Sir Stephen, he was another older heterosexual dominant male with a slave woman at home. But this slave master had a JCPenney wardrobe, plus the stiff posture, clipped diction and dead serious attitude which screamed ex-military. "I will not tolerate willful disobedience," barked Master Peter, as he ran his open hand through his close-cropped head of almost hair. "If you don't make rules, and don't tell them what to do, the slave will not be fulfilled. Owners must also enforce, follow up on their rules. A slave must not say 'this is how it should be'; the master must say 'this is what I need.' But keep in mind there must be some compatibility. You must take into account a slave's interests and desires. And ask yourself how far you want to take it. Do you want to push for a Total Power Exchange or go somewhere near vanilla? Because the line is where *you* draw it."

I thought about Clive, with his fixed ideas of what slavery is and isn't. He had even objected to my use of *relationship*, a word I'd heard during the Master/slave workshop with regularity. "*Ahem!*" Clive had cleared his throat in a sarcastic, annoying way. "Owners don't have a relationship with their slave, they merely have an ownership association."

It was nearly lunchtime and as a closing remark, Master Peter spoke of the need to compromise. "Also keep in mind, some potential owners have spent the past five years of their lives looking for their slave, because that master just can't compromise."

The uncompromisingly picky Manhattan male, was he also among the ranks of slave owners? I chatted with such a guy all through our nearly gourmet, undeniably edible box lunch. During the morning's lectures, he'd been hard to ignore: sitting next to me was the most attractive man in the room.

Looking much like a male model, this tall, tan and fit fellow had a fine head of dark hair and was dressed in the sleek, casual elegant style I had suggested Bradley adopt. Master GQ wore an expensive looking, beautifully tailored, well-fitting range of blacks and charcoals, all in exquisite taste. As he ate the catered meal, I glanced at his shoes, remembering how my girlfriends had long proclaimed you could tell a man's financial status this way. These were absolutely the most perfect pair of Italian made thin-soled shoes a dude could don to enslave a lady. His name tag read Master Ryan* and he appeared to be either a trader, big time broker or investment banker.

"I love what you're wearing," I complimented him. "Where do you shop for your clothes?"

"I'm wearing Armani but Paul Stuart also seems to satisfy my needs."

"I wish I could get my slave to dress as you do. But I'm not here because of any problems with *him*," I clarified. "I'm trying to figure out my deal with another slave, this unruly English slave."

"An English slave, huh. You mistresses seem to have a surfeit of slaves. Me, I'm having a hard time finding just *one*," he responded, with more than a tinge of bitterness.

"Someone like you? How can that be?" I blurted.

Eligible middle aged single men have now come to confide in me (the much older woman beyond the realm of romantic possibility) how they "can't find what they're looking for" which is, typically, a head turner with an advanced degree, and from a wealthy family. Oh, there's also how she has to be beautiful "on the inside and out." With Master Ryan it was the same old song, but with a twist.

"I just can't seem to find the right slave," he complained. "Sure, I've been with plenty of submissive women. A *ton* of them. I'm here to sharpen my command of power and control so I can find exactly what I'm looking for. But it's not easy."

"So, what kind of scene are you seeking?" I was curious to learn what kink had enthralled him.

"I'm a dom, naturally and het definitely—but not really fixated on any one activity. I just can't seem to find..." As he paused, his placid, conventionally handsome face took on more character, suddenly contorted by the depth of his emotion, longing and frustration. "I can't seem to get a girl who has—one: a real bubbly personality. Two: a high level job. And three: wants me to tie her up and whip her. It's just always," he sighed, "as if one of those elements is missing."

Even kinksters have their laundry list. "Well, that shouldn't be such a tall order," I replied, trying to seem positive.

Master Ryan placed his elbows on the table and leaned his head into his open hands, as if genuinely distraught, before he continued. "It's not about needing the supermodel, that's not my thing. But I must have a woman who runs the show at her workplace during the day. These women are out there, I know. I'm always getting fixed up with them. But they usually don't have a certain giggly, cheerleader quality I find such a turn on. They're too fucking serious, and just so stressed out. That kind of boss lady, well she just doesn't know how to act around a guy, like your basic stripper knows how to handle herself. I mean a dancer—they call themselves *dancers*. She's not a man and she knows it!"

"So you've never met one top level professional woman who knows how to act like a cheerleader, even if she's been one in high school?"

"Not really."

"Then why don't you go out with a stripper? They make plenty of money."

"I need someone who's in my league."

"But with a bubbly personality and eager to be bound, gagged and whipped?"

"No gags—I get off on the vocals. But basically, that's it." He slumped in his seat. "I think I'll always be alone," he muttered.

Sir Stephen approached. "Ah, Mistress Pussycat. Are you comfortable in this chair?"

"I certainly am, it's very well padded. Thank you for bringing it in just for me." While others sat in metal edged office chairs, Sir Stephen seemed attentive to my needs and had provided me with what I required.

"And are you getting something out of the workshop?"

"Yes, there's lots being said I needed to hear. But my situation is so strange."

"Oh, how so?" I now stood up and faced him so he could better hear me, without any sordid details possibly being overheard by others.

"I wrote you how this English slave was soon coming over for inspection and a trial period. Well, he's very odd, wanting to be naked and shackled. Now this fellow insists he sleep while wearing chains. Chains! He says keeping him restrained makes him feel safe and secure."

"Slave Marianne!" Sir Stephen called abruptly, in the direction of the nearby kitchen. "You *must* join us now." The woman dropped her dishtowel and scurried over to her master's side. "Please tell Mistress Pussycat when and how we met."

"It was in 1999, about a dozen years ago. We met online in a chat room for masters to hook up with slaves," she stated.

"So you'd never met before you came to live with Sir Stephen?"

"Never met him. We'd just exchanged pictures, talked on the phone, and then I moved halfway across the country to be his slave."

"Slave Marianne, tell her how you wanted to appear when you first arrived."

"Oh, in those days it was no clothes for me, not inside the house. I wanted to be naked and in chains. Had to have those chains!" she laughed merrily while remembering. "But I got over it. Once I experienced the thrill of having my fantasy fulfilled, I didn't need to be naked and in chains anymore. It got in the way of my duties."

"You see, Mistress Pussycat? Slaves seem extreme at first, and may have very specific fantasies. But they'll get over it." Sir Stephen elucidated.

"I suppose you're right. But Clive's different, and says he's a *born slave*, one created specifically to be owned."

"But there's no predestined genetic code for a *born* slave. They're just slaves."

"There's no such thing as a born slave?" I repeated with the dull acceptance of an eight-year-old having been told the truth about Santa. "This guy insists he's not even human but a separate hybrid species of subhumanoid, a product of genetic mutation and natural selection. Seriously! He says he's been studied by scientists or biologists and he's been classified not as *Homo sapiens* but *Homo mancipium*."

At this, both Sir Stephen and his slave broke out in laughter. "Clever guy, huh?" he added. "I know where he got that. The term *mancipium* was used during the Roman Empire. They were not exactly a slave, but a free man under the control of a Roman family. A mancipium couldn't be abused or killed without cause, unlike a Roman slave. You must already know how slaves, unlike subs, have very strong personalities. They are very opinionated, not meek in the least. You'll find any slave is pretty much the control freak. Right?" he beamed down at slave Marianne, who was also smiling. "For you to manage someone with such a dominant personality, well, it may be a struggle at first. But you must treat them as you would a servant. Because if you don't, they will quickly lose respect. And instead of service, all you'll receive is their contempt."

This was totally in keeping with what Clive had been telling me. "You must also determine what is core, or essential to your needs," Sir Stephen continued. "I thought I needed my first meal of the day to be served at five o'clock, when I rise. But slave Marianne needs eight hours of sleep and maybe more. I determined her health was more important than having her get me my early morning coffee. So she sleeps in a bit while I breakfast on my own. You have to make adjustments in the best interest of your slave. There's other areas, though, where there's just no meeting of the minds. You'll find it difficult to balance maintaining control and also compromise. So if you need mentoring, we're here for you. Right, slave Marianne?"

"It would be my pleasure, Mistress," she replied, before the couple retreated to speak with others.

Perhaps I'd have them over to dinner after Clive arrived. After all, they seemed an ideal couple. He had what he wanted—to live the Victorian lifestyle and have a slave. She'd gotten the life she wanted, to be a slave, while also becoming her master's lawful wedded wife a few years later. The household also had an additional live-in slave, Lisa*, who toiled under slave Marianne the way a parlor maid reported to the head housemaid in Victorian times.

I once asked a married girlfriend, then living in the suburbs, who she thought were the happiest couples—those with both spouses working, or couples where the wife stayed at home. I remembered her wise reply: "Who brings home the bacon doesn't matter. The only happy couples in the suburbs are those who know what their deal is. You'd be surprised at how many are married, but still haven't figured it out."

Sir Stephen and slave Marianne certainly knew what their deal was. And I knew there was no deal to be had with Bradley and the suburbs, his spawn, his service bottom needs. What could possibly be my deal with Clive? I'll torture and control him if he pampers and takes care of me? Both relationship were certifiably bizarre—yet I'd observed many marriages founded on a bedrock of far worse behaviors.

Sir Stephen announced workshops were resuming with the topic of Leadership presented by Sir Richard*, who'd been active in the BDSM arena for over a decade. According to the Armani clad Master Ryan, Sir Richard was the group's historian, with an intriguing personal history. Clean-cut, good looking Richard appeared to be the typical prosperous young professional who held down a responsible corporate position. He lived in a sizable dwelling with his wife (who was also successful) and young kids; all benefited from the respectful ministrations of three to four well-trained servants. When it came to those women who have little children plus big careers, I'd heard others admiringly say: "I don't know how she does it all." This couple decided to forgo the day-care option, forget the paid live-in help—just get a bunch of stone kinksters to do their shopping, cleaning and childcare. While Sir Richard and his wife toiled at their impressive jobs, I wondered whether they used a Nanny Cam to spy on their unpaid household helpers.

Sir Richard's afternoon lecture described how he runs his household. This encompassed rules utilized by nobility's low-level domestics in eras past as well as present day bottom-rank Army enlistees. Although Sir Richard was very active in this masters-of-slaves group, he always described those who served him as *servants*, and treated them as exactly that.

There were actually two masters in his household (Sir Richard and his wife Lady Beth*) both to be obeyed. These masters' requirements and requests were the primary, constant focus for their slaves. And there were plenty who desired to be useful to this couple. With an extensive interview and vetting process, Sir Richard had to turn away most of the many seeking to serve. They all held down responsible jobs—he selected only those having a useful skill or organizational ability. I could only imagine how Sir Richard's kids would rationalize it, after realizing they're neither immensely wealthy nor descended from royalty, yet had several servants attending them. Was Sir Richard's lifestyle beyond typical scandalous *Jerry Springer Show* territory or an unconventional yet viable option to more conventional choices such as cleaning ladies and au pair girls? The bowing and scraping, the multiple minions toiling at the bequest of their masters within the confines of a home—it all must have resembled an extreme college fraternity house pledge period, a perpetual Hell Week. But for those men and women with an inner need to be controlled, their nirvana awaited at Chez Richard.

Sir Richard was expert in protocol, which details how one must treat their servants, proper slave behavior, plus the rituals in which both slaves and owners take part. He was also well versed in the history of consensual slavery, as it developed in America.

Modern consensual slavery (specifically, its practice in the United States) began as a by-product of the modern BDSM scene, which in turn sprang from the homosexual leather community. Psychotherapist and BDSM expert Guy Baldwin, in his 1993 book *Ties That Bind*, explains how gay U.S. servicemen in World War II triumphantly returned home after experiencing brutal wartime combat overseas, yet missed that special mix of hierarchy, brotherhood and testosterone they'd found so intense, especially in the face of danger. These gay former soldiers founded an organized leather community which emphasized their butch sexuality. At that time, the macho gay man was an unfamiliar aspect of homosexuality, as opposed to the more commonly known feminine, foppish "pansy."

These leather folk found expression in studs, chains, motorcycles, biker's caps, and the ubiquitous black leather. Yet another phenomenon initially created by gays and ultimately adopted by heterosexuals, consensual slavery's proclivity for rules—plus punishments for breaking them—indirectly evolved from enlisted men's experience in the U.S. Armed Forces.

"Say, were there any high-powered women there?" Bradley asked much later, over dinner.

"Maybe there were one or two businesswomen types at the workshop; but I couldn't tell how successful they were. The group seemed be to be from a cross section of society. Wall Streeters. Preppy corporate types. Fashionable, well-groomed older women alongside the leather-clad bull dyke. They were all different and all just regular people like us!"

While we dined, we were asked if everything was to our satisfaction. Oh, it was—what a *nouvelle cuisine* feast! The waiter had shot us his approving look for the attractive older couple—the man still out with one who was obviously his first wife.

"Are you glad you went, Mistress?" asked Bradley as he sipped his wine.

"Certainly. I not only learned a lot, I got to see The Real Slaves Of New York."

Later in the evening, I was inspired to set up a little scene for the domination deprived Bradley. Although I was a bit drunk, I made him place his penis in a rope's slipknot and led him around my apartment. Then, while he was stationary on all fours, I placed one foot on his back, while still wearing my high heeled sandals. Bradley had given me a pedicure and painted my toenails the weekend before—he loved caring for my feet. As expected, he responded well to the foot-on-slave victory pose. I fell asleep wondering why I'd never pulled the rope trick on Bradley before.

A much satisfied Bradley slept on my living room sofa bed. I closed my bedroom door and settled in for a full night's slumber, the cats nestled beside me, before a phone call awakened me at eight o'clock the next morning. Slave Clive was on the line, anxious to hear what was discussed at the Master/slave Development Center workshop. "It's too early, let's talk later," I mumbled.

"Rubbish! It's afternoon here and I've waited all bloody day to hear how that New York slavery group would regard a born slave such as myself." Clive had once agreed to use the video chat at a local internet cafe but found it too inconvenient, so he always telephoned. According to Bradley, Clive seemed to call me way too often.

"Well, one of the many things they mentioned was how there's no such thing as a *born slave*. According to them, you are absolutely 100 percent human and slaves aren't genetically or biologically different."

"You paid proper pounds to hear such utter nonsense? Exactly who told you this bald-faced lie?" slave Clive raged.

"The founder of the Master/slave Development Center himself and a foremost expert on consensual slavery, Sir Stephen."

"*Sir* Stephen?" repeated Clive, in an indignant tone. "Well, fancy that! The chap dares to call himself such when he has most certainly not been knighted? Not Viscount, Earl, Marquis or Duke Stephen? Frankly, I don't give a red cents damn what the so-called slavery organizations say. I know I am a slave and also a human hybrid species! Though outwardly human, my internal organs are anatomically atypical. I may think and behave differently. My brain wave patterns are quite unusual as well. And I make no apologies for that," he huffed.

My bedroom door was open and Bradley now entered. *"Ugh*, slave Clive," he groaned, having heard my end of the conversation. I nodded to him, all the while holding the telephone receiver far away in my outstretched arm. I chose not to hear the invective my prospective slave was spewing far over the Atlantic. "I'm going to check on my car," Bradley whispered before leaving.

I responded to slave Clive calmly, continuing my report of the day's events. "After inspection, Stephen noted the probationary period should not be a set period of time, but day to day. And he offered to mentor me, to check in with us and see how the slavery was coming along. He was such a great guy," I enthused. "And I thought I hated all dominant males..."

My potential slave cut me off. "Madam, have you taken even one bloody second to consider *my* needs?"

"Of course I have—you are constantly reminding me of them."

"How would I eat?"

"You'd eat the same healthy, nutritious foods I do. And you'd cook them as well."

"Now, madam, exactly where would I eat such food? At some wretched kitchen table set with china or out of a dog bowl on the kitchen floor?"

"I hadn't thought of it, actually."

"Seems as if you haven't thought of a lot—like where you would keep me when I'm not being used."

"I have several rugs, there are sofas and chairs."

"When not in service, a slave should be attached by a chain to a ring on the wall. Or locked in his cage."

"Where would I put a cage, Clive? I have only one bedroom, and you're not messing up my living room!"

"That's *slave* Clive, madam, and not only do I have a five-bedroom home nearby, I keep a cage there. Sad to say, it is not really my ideal cage; but I am sending you a link to what I consider the perfect cage. If you approve of the dimensions, I'll order it at once. My return to the States is imminent and I must prepare for my true vocation. Towards that end," he cleared his throat before continuing, "I shall also order a newer model milking machine which should keep me in tip-top condition."

"A milking machine? You mean a blender to make smoothies? I already have a juicer."

"No, no, no! When a male is in *chas-ti-ty*," (Clive always drew out this word and also *slavery*, emphasizing every syllable to give it extra importance) "he should receive regular milking to maintain good hygiene." (Yet more kinky behavior cloaked as healthy living.) "Milking helps flush out the toxins which accumulate within the prostate gland of a chaste male."

"No way am I giving a prostate massage to you or anyone else!"

"Nor should you, madam. You must let the milking machine do it!"

"They have a machine for just about everything these days, don't they? Is this similar to the dairy farm devices that get attached to old Bessie's udders?"

"You needn't be snide concerning practices about which you've absolutely no understanding. A milking session may last ten minutes or so, until the slave begins to release fluid, which becomes property of the key holder. Perhaps it is collected in a cup or saucer as it dribbles down. A strict key holder will insist you consume your own ejaculate as demonstration of your slave status, proof positive you are humble."

As Bradley re-entered my apartment, I hissed into the phone: "slave Clive, you need correction! Catch you later." I then hung up on him.

I later checked my e-mail and clicked on a link Clive had sent. There were pictures plus instructions for a product called the Slavemate. The manufacturer noted its product was versatile enough to be used in countless imaginative ways—as spreaders or a collar set, for restraint, kneeling, even as a bending over device. They promised all the tools and attachment any master or mistress could possibly ever need, but offered this warning: "Do not leave your slave unattended."

Was this really the only choice I had, between these two guys? With Clive there would surely be a cage in the living room. But Bradley and his daughter promised something even worse—a playpen. After Bradley's return to suburbia the next day, I received a call from a predictably peeved Clive. I had long realized the man I knew as slave Clive was clearly not in his right mind, though this was why I was so fascinated by him. He was a one-of-a-kind kind of guy.

"I am most certainly not pleased, madam. Not in the least. It seems as if you've been rather critical and also negatively humorous towards me. You further antagonized me by hanging up when I merely inquired how you were getting on. The cheek of it! Now I'm soon returning to a life unfulfilled, as I shall be totally adrift without an owner. Madam, you've dashed my destiny!"

"You needn't be so critical and negative, slave Clive. I agreed to meet you and promised we'd then discuss a trial arrangement."

"*Bah*, your submissive boyfriend would never agree. If you want access to his dosh you must pander to his needs. And they don't include having any naked slaves in chastity and shackles about!"

"Probably not. But who says I want to be with Bradley or even need access to his...what's your word for money, *dosh*? What if I have my own dosh and don't want to live in a house with him and his brood?"

"If that's the case, perfectly splendid, madam. I will strive to improve your daily existence and make you proud. I do hope with time, you'll come to view slave ownership as natural, if a bit underground. You see, there are a few groups of women who own slaves, support each other and even trade slaves. These women are difficult to locate though, due to their secrecy. Most of them have elevated careers and positions in society."

There it was again, the submissive man's fetishistic reverence for high-powered women. "I met no such female slave owners at the workshop; but that doesn't mean they aren't out there."

"Precisely, madam, and why I suggest you do some networking. Now, if you agree, I'm going to forward you some links to a few female owners I've noticed online who seem like they'd make good mentors for you. Get some ideas from them."

"Seems to me you're just chock full of ideas yourself, slave Clive."

"Simply review how they present themselves, take notice of their lifestyle and what they're looking for in a slave. Then, when I call you tomorrow, I'd be most interested in hearing your thoughts."

That evening I booted up my computer to find the women Clive would have me emulate. The first lady owner neither profiled nor displayed a picture of herself, but instead listed the name of her land, O-Beat-ient-Ranch*. Both she and her husband were willing to whip, flog and anally penetrate dedicated masochists in exchange for free ranch work. It appeared as if they already had themselves a crew of willing victims down on the farm, yet were looking for more.

The second role model, a very plump redhead, showed herself within the confines of her home office. She had started her own business (again with her husband) and lived in the Deep South. The typical laundry list of fetishes fulfilled was offered by this dominant goddess, who also specified her slave must have both computer knowledge and office skills. The third owner was more vague about why she wanted a slave, but noted she was a domme who was married to a dom.

"I may not be an expert on slavery, but those women want to own slaves for all the wrong reasons," I declared when Clive called the next day. "How can a domme be married to a *dom*? If they're together, how much power and control can she exercise? She probably submits to her husband!"

"Indeed, how utterly disagreeable," he replied in a subdued tone.

"And the redhead with a home business. Let her hire someone who works for a living wage, and not rely on BDSM for free labor. The chick's so fat she probably thinks Crisco is one of the five food groups. And don't get me started about the Brokeback Mountain brigade down at the ranch. Guys mending fences, herding cattle and hauling hay just so they can get their regular back-whipping, ass-poking endorphin high. These women you look up to as role models aren't dommes or owners—they're *users*!"

"Quite right, madam. You are simply what you are. And I believe you will make one excellent success of being a real slave owner, but in your own individual and unique manner."

As we finished our conversation, I realized I'd made Clive see things my way. I felt a sense of pride and accomplishment, as if through continuous effort I'd somehow tamed a wild horse—one I was willing to ride.

FOURTEEN

Two Slaves Too Many

BRADLEY, WEARING ONLY A TOWEL WRAPPED around his waist, entered my bedroom. "I've done my slave grooming and pretty much butchered my nipples with the razor. Do you have any Band-Aids, Mistress?"

Men who are consensual slaves (or in Bradley's case, think of themselves as such) often shave their chest or genitals hairless. I only glanced at his bleeding pecs. "They're in the lower shelf above the toilet," I muttered. I was ready to switch slaves and trade in this grandpa for someone more interesting. Would it be Clive, who would soon return stateside? That was doubtful, as slave Clive now wanted to turn his suburban home into some sort of BDSM resort.

"Sophisticated women could use my home as a private place where they can enjoy dominating men. For the gents, bedrooms will be furnished with cages, a St. Andrew's Cross, and whipping benches. For the ladies, a bed and dressing table will suffice. The women must be female supremacists who firmly believe all men are inferior to them, without exception. So, you see, my home would become your home, too."

I was reaching retirement age and owned a cozy, one-bedroom co-op in Chelsea. There was also a comfortable nest egg, one to make this old bird think twice before flying the coop. What kind of future living arrangements were each of these men offering me? There would be Bradley's country place to be filled with other people's children, or Clive's suburban domicile, possibly the ultimate house which is not a home.

I had explained to slave Clive: "Bradley satisfies my needs for companionship and social things like restaurants, art galleries, theater and museums. This is what ladies love and a good part of why I live in Manhattan. But he cannot offer me an acceptable living situation because he does not have control over his kid—the kid has control of him. And I can say this about many men I know, not just Bradley."

"Mistress, shall I draw you a bath?" asked Bradley as he reappeared, four or five Band-Aids now affixed to his chest.

"According to Clive, a slave should wear a hood with no cut-out for the eyes when bathing his mistress. He says it's how slaves bathed their owners in the Middle Ages." Bradley, who was rapidly growing jealous, could tell I was fascinated by Clive.

"Oh, he sounds like a real poster boy for sanity," Bradley mumbled.

"And I suppose your Doctor Domme is a paragon of mental health."

We soon left, with my cats in their carriers, for Bordello Park, the name Bradley had given a lush garden near the West Chelsea discos, where hookers took their johns in the early morning hours. We sat on benches among the plants, trees and flowers, each of us holding and stroking a leashed cat. Their nostrils trembled as they breathed the verdant scents and their necks stretched towards the sun. People looking in would think we were a compatible pair of cat lovers.

When most couples get together, there is a meeting of the minds and making of space, changes which involve more than a few sacrifices. The prospect of having a slave in the place of a mate seemed to be an appealing lifestyle choice—just not with Bradley. One of the Bordello Park bushes had a used condom draped around a rose well past full bloom. "Tell me, think you'd ever want to get married one day?" he asked.

"I've put marriage in the same category as organized religion and anal sex—not for me."

"I don't know if I can see you next weekend," he replied.

"Doctor Domme needs you, I suppose?"

"Oh, no, if that were the case I would definitely know one way or the other, then ask your permission. I just don't know because it's my older grandson's birthday and I had promised my daughter I'd take them all to the beach. But the visitation with her ex-husband still has to be worked out. Then again, my daughter could have to put in some time at the store. I don't want to take her kids to the beach without her. They're toddlers. And such a handful!"

"O.K., it's complicated. We shouldn't make plans for next weekend," I suggested.

"But maybe I can come down to see you. I'll let you know right after both my daughter and son-in-law find out if they're working. It all depends on whether the daughter of the old lady my son-in-law takes care of on weekends can be with her mother next weekend. If that old lady's grandchild doesn't need the daughter, then my daughter's ex-husband takes custody for the weekend with no visitation, so no beach. He'll let us know the day before."

"I'd rather not be left hanging when I can make other plans."

"Would these other plans include slave Clive?"

"They may, as he is soon returning to his New Jersey home. I would want to meet such a dedicated slave in person." Bradley, who often gazed at me obliquely, when not actively training his eyes to be cast downward, shot me a direct, knowing and somewhat accusatory look. My eyes met his as I wished he could read my mind: *I would rather spend time with a man who wore a chastity belt, shackles and chains than someone whose life was controlled by his child's ex-husband's client's granddaughter.*

Much later in the evening, slave Clive called me, excited by his home improvement plans. "We'll create a female supremacy utopia and refuge, but the women must be naturally cautious and secretive to protect each other," he advised. "It can be staffed by the inferior male entities who come to serve the mistresses. My place sleeps eight people and if cages are placed in some rooms, a dozen people can be easily accommodated."

"Sounds like Other World Kingdom is relocating to just across the

Hudson River."

"Quite so, Mistress. The women must exercise proper physical and emotional control over the males by discipline, degradation and humiliation. They must demand their submissives be subject to celibacy. Plus, they can claim ownership of a male, either formally or informally. You'd be headmistress, firmly in charge."

"Oh, I truly do doubt that."

"Don't tell me you'd prefer being with your namby-pamby Mr. B.!"

"No, slave Clive. Among your attributes is the fact you have no kids who run and ruin your life."

"Were you to be my mistress, I would worship you as a living goddess. You see, madam, I want, I need to be *owned*," he replied in a dramatic, throaty voice.

I had discovered how many potential or former slaves have a driving need to be owned. But the *ronin*, or orphan slave, was a BDSM phenomenon which disturbed me. I could have this morbid curiosity about (or sometimes feel compassion for) many subs, even the oddest fetishist. But when it came to a *ronin*, as was the slave Ralph with whom I'd spoken, a rage emerged to match my sympathy. It appeared as though Ralph's owner had faked her own death and sent him to a remote motel, where he toiled wage-free. How could some irresponsible dominant woman take a man, break the man and leave him helpless to fend for himself? And were there as many *ronin* among the ranks of submissive female slaves, women who were cast aside by doms and left homeless after years of domestic servitude, perhaps because they had aged? I suspected as much, yet actually had no idea.

One such male *ronin* confessed he was now living on the streets of Manhattan. I shouldn't have even met him, but the picture he'd sent had haunted me. In his early thirties, athletically built and white bread handsome, his hands were wrapped around two bars of the metal cage which contained him. Apart from his tats and piercings, he had the conventional All American Boy look. I wondered how he'd come to be in that cage and whether it was something he actually wanted, as Clive had claimed about himself.

I met the All American Boy for coffee. He was tall, if a bit scruffy, as attractive as his picture, and carried a track cell phone, where you pay by the minute. It was the perfect phone service plan for those who had no one to call and nowhere to go. The guy had severed many ties during his ten years of service (I'd call it captivity) having lost touch with family and old friends. He confided he was ashamed to relate what had happened to him for the past decade. According to him, no one would ever understand how the All American Boy could wind up homeless, so emotionally shattered, all because he was in thrall to a dominant woman who'd eventually abandoned him. He didn't have a life apart from being her slave—submission took over his very being. This mistress had programmed her All American Boy so completely, after she left he felt he'd no real life.

This All American Boy had never worked a regular job, just a few stints waiting tables at restaurants. He'd dropped out of college to live in New York, an ideal place to try breaking through as an actor. It was tough going, unlike his small Midwestern home town where he'd been every bit the big deal—star athlete, popular, cock of the walk. In New York City, no longer bolstered by his hometown reputation, he found the competition tough and landing acting gigs near impossible. His ego took the inevitable beating. Through an acting class, he met the woman to whom he became enslaved. She wasn't a prostitute, he revealed, as he hungrily finished one sandwich, then another (he must have been starving) but worked as a pro-domme. After having lived together for nearly ten years, she had left town permanently, and without her slave. On hearing about his current nowhere-to-go problem, I paid for his food, gave him what was left in my wallet (only two twenties), wished him the best of luck, and went on my way. Though slave Clive was possibly certifiable, at least he seemed self-sufficient. The All American Boy, besides being young enough to be my son, was not for me. A pathetic case, he was seeking a new home and owner in lieu of a life.

I'd been contacted by a few dominant women owners who were trying to find a new home for their slave. One was a local lesbian couple who wanted to "dispose of and situate" their male live-in. I spoke to the *femme*, who described her partner as "more of a dyke." The fellow was left to them by a domme who had died the year before and asked that her slave be given to a woman who sought real ownership, not just a BDSM play pal. The dear departed had taught the man how his enslavement is the foundation of happiness and emphasized how pleasing his mistress is not just a job, but his bliss. The lesbian couple had kept the man, who was in his fifties, naked and shackled, as their friend had.

The woman tried to sell me on her slave's usefulness—how he cheerfully cleaned the apartment, cooked, and was good with repairs. Just when this began to sound like someone trying to get work for their underemployed cleaning lady, she added: "He will lick a clit and never seems to get tired of it. Of course, you don't have to pleasure him back. But I think it's fun to make him rub himself while he's on his knees making love to my feet, worshipping my toes."

I asked why she was getting rid of him. "I'm part of a lesbian couple, and we're just not very kinky," she explained. "So we're not really enjoying him as much as a dominant heterosexual woman would. Why don't you talk to him. You can examine him and then, if you want to own him, he has no choice!"

I explained I had a slave arriving soon from England and wished her luck placing the guy. Responsible owners will always take care of their slave and have a sincere interest in his wellbeing. They house him, provide food and clothing plus cover all medical expenses. The worst thing an owner could do would be to leave their slave a *ronin*, or a slave without an owner.

Mistress Roberta*, who had entered matrimony *sans* baggage, didn't want to make a *ronin* of Thog*, her devoted slave. In the way one cat lover reaches out to another about a certain deserving abandoned feline, asking if anyone knows of a good home, mistresses seek out those like-minded about slavery. But they first determine whether the future owner candidate is even qualified, ever mindful there are many degrees of ownership, from casual to the most severe.

As I was active in several consensual slavery groups, I was contacted about Thog, a forty-something male molded to serve and suffer under the strictest of mistresses. According to Mistress Roberta, her slave was "submitted to OWK for a week or more"; but because of his recalcitrant behavior, Thog's time there was prolonged to three weeks. She declared at Other World Kingdom, Thog learned to "respect its superiors and all women." In doing so, he lost almost twenty pounds. But, as she suggested, Thog knew he wasn't boarding Czech Air for any vacation.

I imagined she and Clive were on the same page about slavery, and wanted to learn more. When I called her to ask about the man, she informed me he's not accustomed to being seen as a *man*. "It is not a human being but a *chattel* of his mistress, like livestock," she explained in a crisp, businesslike way. "If allowed to speak, it is not permitted to use words like *me*, *I* or *mine* under threat of severe punishment. It should only speak about itself in third person."

"Can you give me an example?"

"This slavish brute admits to violating rules of behavior by engaging in thought and begs for disciplinary action."

"And what would the punishment be, what's *it* used to?"

"Oh, it is considerably hypersensitive. Torture of its nipples, little cock and testicles makes it writhe wildly. And when in bondage, it is petrified by application of an anti-inflammatory on its genitalia and anus. This is a salve so painful, it can't control itself for over thirty minutes, at least. But I used large gags to quiet down unnecessary noises. We had a downstairs neighbor."

"And what do you get out of this?"

"It was thrilling just for me to witness it consumed in such a frenzied fit—watching the creature squirm, wiggle and twist while hanging on a chain."

She wasn't the first dyed-in-the-wool sadist I'd spoken to. "Ever give it a break?" I hated to sound flippant, but often do when genuinely alarmed.

"Not when it is being penalized. To forgive promised discipline makes it think the owner is weak and can be manipulated. This always results in insubordination, idle behavior and ultimately contempt." She further explained how the owner must be strict and consistent, enforce all rules and punish any violations of behavior. According to her, the slave would be constantly testing his master. I'd heard this before, both from slave Clive and Sir Stephen. It was now becoming apparent that having a slave didn't equal a duty-free life—it was actually a hell of a lot of work.

Mistress Roberta also exercised bastinade as correctional punishment. I knew how bastinade, or beating on bare soles—done usually with sticks—was an OWK favored practice, one as regularly doled out at that Czech-side S&M retreat as goulash, cabbage and dumplings.

"Of course, being in torment breaks it down even more," she added. Mistress Roberta emphasized how Thog was trained to have zero sense of self-esteem. She stressed how it was important for such a slave, while in service training, to cease thinking for himself. For example, Thog was encouraged to repeat out loud certain phrases like "the beast must obey."

As every Roman soldier once had his sword and shield, every hardcore slave apparently wore collar and cuffs, often with leg shackles. Thog was kept in a collar with an attached leash plus a pair of ankle cuffs. (The latter item had a mere one-foot chain restraint, allowing movement only for ordered work.) He was made to wear a rubber or latex partial hood, as his owner confided she didn't like looking at his face and such head gear served to dehumanize him even more.

She'd often insert a butt plug or dildo in her slave's rectum. I wondered exactly what Thog got out of their deal, and asked if her slave had been used for sex. "Of course, any mistress has to train it for her specific bodily needs. It has been utilized as a pleasure toy and actually adds a certain wanton, libidinous feeling about the house. A vibrator in its mouth makes it more functional. But there has never been even a hint of familiarity or attachment. The thing is just like my vibrator—I can turn it on or shut it off merely by moving my index finger."

She only had to lift one finger to make her slave perform as automatically as her electronic equipment. "Usually, just signaling with my finger or uttering a single syllable it heard many times is enough. You see, it is instructed to execute set slave conduct without any autonomous reasoning. Any measure it takes is an automatic response to my orders. But now its new owner must initiate new protocols and control its thinking in her own manner to suit herself. And then," she promised in a more enthusiastic voice, one of a salesperson, "as a result of my disciplinary actions, you'll own a totally subservient domestic creature!"

Some women have likened male behavior modification to training one's dog, though Mistress Roberta's rules make a dog's life seem a comparatively fine one. And just as some pets are not allowed to sit on the furniture, neither was Mistress Roberta's slave. He was also forbidden to eat in the presence of his mistress unless it was for her amusement—for instance, seeing him beg for food or lick his meal out of a dog bowl.

Thog's living quarters were around twenty square feet, while he was not in what his mistress termed "active use." The man she called "it" had, for several years, existed in a certain corner where he was expected to retreat on command. There he would await his owner's new orders, for further use or whatever punishment she meted out. At such times, he was expected to present himself with arms raised and eyes directed at his mistress's feet. When awaiting orders, Mistress Roberta expected her slave's entire body to be at full attention with no movement allowed, not even the licking of dry lips.

And those slave lips were guaranteed to be dry as the Kalahari Desert—drinking water was not part of the program. Consuming what she referred to as her "golden nectar" was offered instead. The man was allowed to drink water from his dog bowl—but mainly while cleaning the mistress's shoes and boots with his tongue.

I had asserted (at a few meetings and on some message boards) I was a dominant woman willing to explore slavery. Although I was only interested in slavery lite, I encouraged the woman to reveal more. "I understand about the punishment, but don't quite get the reward. How have you rewarded it—other than allowing him to drink your urine?"

She sighed. "The reward is to be in the presence, service and training of its owner," she replied, as if speaking to a dullard who just didn't get it.

It was clear (to both of us) I was hardly cut out to be a strict owner, and would have trouble handling such a slave. "He, I mean, *it* sounds great—but very demanding, like a lot of responsibility."

"It isn't a burden," she clarified. "It has a demanding job and is highly successful in its field."

I'd heard it before: master by day, slave by night. Why should I be surprised? "But you left to get married. I thought you were finding a mistress for your slave so he won't be homeless."

"It will be a *ronin*, but hardly homeless. Its name is on the lease of a most accommodating space. As I've mentioned, I now live elsewhere with my new husband. But you're apparently not interested." As we said our good lucks and goodbyes, I could only wonder who the hell she had married!

So Thog wasn't some sort of helpless creature after all—at least, not in his work-a-day life. But for a dedicated submissive slave to become a *ronin*, such an event would pretty much unmoor him. In BDSM, *ronin* refers to a slave without an owner. The word is literally interpreted as wave man, suggesting a transitory state, and originally described either a vagrant or wanderer in feudal Japan. It first referred to those downtrodden hoe-toting serfs who had fled their master's land, not to any fierce sword slinging samurai. But by Edo period Japan, a *ronin* came to mean *samurai* with no lord or master, due to the death or downfall of that superior. And when the Master met his Maker, a samurai's code would have him commit *hara kiri* (ritual suicide). If this integral part of the code was not obeyed, the samurai was shamed and cast aside, destined to spend the rest of his days adrift and alone as a *ronin*. Oddly enough (even for such an odd place as modern Japan) either a Japanese salaryman between jobs or a high school grad awaiting admittance to college is currently called a *ronin*.

I wondered whether the punishment Roberta meted out to Thog was the kind of treatment slave Clive fantasized about and expected. Obviously, he wanted to be controlled; conversely, he was totally uncontrollable. Shortly after speaking with Mistress Roberta, Clive called me in a manic panic about his suburban home and how he'd make it a play space for dominant women and submissive men. Again he threw out a line to reel me in: "My home can be your home, too. Fifty-fifty. But you would have absolute authority there."

"O.K., if that's the case, I'd like to turn the place into a haven for *ronin*, slaves without an owner. Slaves without a home. Slaves in transition who seek either a new mistress, a new master if they're female or gay, or anyone who needs help towards a new submission-free life if they're over being owned."

"And exactly what, madam, has created this one hundred and eighty degree turnaround on your part?" he inquired, in the tone of a snippy butler.

I told him about Mistress Roberta's quest to find a new owner for her slave. Clive was silent, for once, as I detailed her dehumanizing punishment-reward system. "I don't have to explain anything more," I added. "Simply put, I'd rather your sizable home become a way station instead of a whipping station. That's what I'd prefer, what I find necessary, and what I need you, as my slave, to do for me."

"What a lot of rubbish!"

I then hung up on him. Why did I ever imagine helping others—those whose needs and fantasies he understood—would bring Clive a sense of purpose and satisfaction? How could I have thought he'd even be grateful for a sane and sensible owner?

About three days later, as though perhaps he'd thought about the situation, slave Clive called me to explain his position. "You see, madam, I believe what you have in mind for my property is not what's required for the treatment of a real slave. And to be frank, you seem far too kind a person to own a slave like myself. What was the point of telling me about Mistress Roberta and her slave? Sad you can't grasp how ownership of a slave permits one to do things you cannot otherwise do to humans."

"But there are several kinds and styles of ownership..." I interjected, before he continued, cutting me off.

"I do not expect, want or need to be treated nicely or with respect. Such things are never, never to be shown a slave," he thundered. "You may find it best to be with a submissive rather than an authentic born slave due to your odd compassion and social conscience." He uttered these last words with such scorn, I could imagine the sneer contorting his face.

I knew he was right, but still felt deeply disappointed. Would we never meet for his inspection or to begin a trial period? No in-house masseur to press his fingers about my aching tendons and fascia? No hooded servant to wash my back in the bath, as they did in the Dark Ages? I wanted to feel superior, to be waited on and catered to. I craved a bit of *Downton Abbey* in my life and told him as much.

Still critical of me, he begged off slave duty. "All real slaves, be they born to the existence or acquire that nonentity during their lives, would resent it if they were not spoken to, thought of and treated as a slave. You are far too moderate a lady to execute the draconian physical chastisement slaves must endure. It would be better all-around if you were a natural cruel and sadistic female supremacy bitch goddess, but you are not. There is no point in pursuing this matter further. You are not sufficiently motivated enough, not are you dominant enough, or severe enough to successfully own a real slave. I will now take my leave of you."

Clive's diatribe shouldn't have surprised me—Sir Stephen had told me much the same. Thinking I'd never again hear from him, Clive called a week later, reminding me he would return to the States in ten days. "Perhaps we can get together to sort things out," be began. "You've been what I call an up and downer. I believe it would benefit you to see real slavery in action."

I was eager to meet and see how we'd interact, as I regarded this man to be the ultimate challenge. "Everything I've decided has been to develop your true nature. But slave Clive, you're a handful and need chastisement!"

"But it seems as if you are anti-chastisement, madam."

"What I don't approve of is when a mistress indoctrinates a guy into slavery then abandons him. I am mainly critical of these dommes' irresponsibility. You have not met or spoken with some of the abandoned slaves, the *ronin*, as I have."

"It seems as though you are both a decent and an honorable woman.

Which is why I want you to meet me in Alabama, where we'll observe a real slave colony in action. Towards that end, I will be booking and paying for two airline tickets. You need this experience, just as I need to be legally owned. And it is perfectly permissible to own a slave since it is not human, and cannot be subject to human laws."

As he spoke in his calm and even persuasive way, I realized he was more than different—more like completely out of his mind. I was always up for taking trips a guy pays for; but certainly not one I've never met, and who insists he's not human. "Look, slave Clive, you'll be in New York next week. We must meet and get acquainted before even thinking of traveling together."

"But we wouldn't be traveling together—I want you to meet me there. It's just for a weekend. Besides visiting the actual slaves, we can tour the nearby plantations and visit the historic old slave quarters. Some of them have preserved the actual shackles and whipping posts!"

"Sounds like an interesting trip." I assumed we'd visit one of the Black slave colonies he'd told me about previously. "But I need to know and feel comfortable around someone first before vacationing with them. That goes for females, males, slaves, and subhuman nonentities alike. Besides, I'm more into touring Charleston or Savannah where they have old Southern homes within a walkable city. Even though I was reared in the South, I'm just not interested in plantations."

"How can you not be fascinated by your ancestors' slaveowner heritage?"

"My grandparents and their grandparents certainly owned no slaves."

"What are you saying, madam? That you are perhaps a naturalized citizen?"

"No, I was born in America. My grandparents came over from Europe in the early twentieth century."

"And where were they from, may I ask?"

During our many conversations, slave Clive had asked very little about me, apart from how I would treat him as a slave. I had not viewed this as a red flag, just a refreshing change from the drill most men delivered: *Where do you work? Who did you marry? Are you family-oriented?*

I imagined slave Clive now wanted to know about my heritage. "I heard my grandparents say they came from Vilnius, which is in Lithuania, but I also learned about a town called Vilna in Poland where a lot of Jews had lived. So it could be either. I think they were too busy with pogroms to think about owning any slaves."

"Don't tell me you are...*a Jew*!" he exclaimed, in a horrified voice.

"Yes, I'm a Southern Jew long settled in New York."

"Christ on a crutch! Forget it, then! There is no trip down South in the offing. They won't take you!"

"You actually think I can't tour Southern plantations because I'm Jewish? Are you really that deranged?"

"The slave colony, madam. They are connected to a church and this just won't do! A pity, that. I must now bid you farewell." He hung up the phone abruptly, forgetting how just a week or two prior, he had proposed worshipping me as a living goddess.

An Anti-Semite, though not a terribly typical one, I cared to hear nothing more from him. His behavior only became clear a day later, after I'd received a message from a dominant woman claiming she resided in the Deep South. A church elder, she'd recently been told I had an interest in joining her dubious denomination. "This is one tall order for the true and devout," she wrote. I assumed slave Clive had his hand in this. A few details were provided and as they say, the Devil is in the details. "Evidence of being in one of the Christian faiths, such as First Communion, confirmation or baptism, will be required from you."

Why was Clive so upset when learning of my religion? Because I wouldn't qualify for his crazy church. I read on. The woman informed me how her subjects are selected, calling it a staged progression and candidate elimination process. It included a tour of the church, face to face meetings, signing of agreements, then "surrendering into voluntary slavery with us for ten years." Now I understood the reason for Clive's sudden proposed trip.

This questionable church lady specified they'd prefer "Christian masochists who seriously wish to combine belief with true service to God and your fellow beings." She added: "Our Elders who govern parochial affairs have instructed me to search for such individuals, as we have witnessed the benefits of genuine cures for a wide range of ailments through the intercession of painful suffering. You must possess a genuine calling for suffering dedicated to the benefit of others' physical wellbeing."

I'd long ago heard of these backwater cults—where terminally ill patients were told how inflicting pain on others will cure their mortal illness or chronic condition—but thought it was a hillbilly version of an urban legend. What Clive had in mind for me seemed an even worse fate than what Bradley proposed—living in a country house with my slave, his daughter and two toddlers.

I was clearly out of my depth, wading about a koi pond of playacting, never diving into the ocean of authentic ownership. Sir Stephen had warned me how a strict, orthodox slave can be contemptuous of, and even turn on a lax mistress. But I hadn't really absorbed his message.

I thought about visiting Charleston and Savannah, only to see how the Old South and New South had combined and evolved, but certainly not with Clive. Whether he was an armchair fantasist or an authentically dangerous madman, I've no idea; I never met him and was well rid of our long distance association. My experience with the man who called himself "slave Clive" made me abandon the D/s lifestyle and take up with a vanilla man whom I had known for decades. But all through that relationship, my thoughts and fantasies revolved around submissive men, despite my previous experience with them.

FIFTEEN

"Let's Be Girls Together"

MY MORNING MIGRAINE WAS LIKE A RATTLESNAKE: it did not strike without warning. On rainy mornings or when the barometric pressure significantly changed, I'd hear a certain rattle within my head; minutes later my brain would begin to spasm. After popping a Zomig, I'd be rid of the headache some twenty minutes later. Prior to my discovering Zolmitriptan, frequent migraines had been debilitating events, and for too many years. Now at 65 and retired, I considered myself lucky to be in good health and not disabled.

The five a.m. walk to the medicine cabinet had dislodged Oedipuss from the curve of my stomach, where he usually slept. Now his sister, Pinky, rose from her usual spot, by my chest, wanting to be fed. I loved being surrounded by my cats and knew of nothing more comforting than this sweet kitty blanket. I'd always found cats to be relaxing but could take people only in small doses.

I was finally finished with the vanilla fellow I'd been dating and ready to re-enter that freak show tent in the submissive circus. A visit to the chiropractor every five weeks kept me pain free. A regular cleaning lady ensured my place was clean and comfortable. Having such an easy life, I no longer desired a slave to kneel, toil and toady...though I'd previously found the prospect strangely appealing. I'd behaved like the irresponsible idiot who fancies getting an exotic pet, all the while knowing how impractical (and possibly dangerous) this would be. Consensual slavery wasn't really about being taken care of; it required too much focus and mindfulness (work!) on the owner's part.

Now awake, I looked at my e-mail, clicking on a message from a Middle Eastern sub:

> *hello. Kiss on Your feet Mistress. Mistress, how can i get a little space close to Your feet? i live in Queens but am originally from Iran. i will worship You and can die for Your pleasure. Your wish will be my command. after making me Your slave You can cut me in pieces and i will not say a single word. 24/7 365 days i can serve You. so please allow me to show my devotion. i will not disappoint You.*
>
> *regards,*
> *slave*

I knew how he must feel. Low. Very low. I'd often thought of the *ronin* like Ralph and the All American Boy, men whose lives had been upended when their mistresses left. I also remembered how the All American Boy had revealed his mistress earned fairly decent money doing financial domination.

When I first investigated femdom, I'd spoken a few times with a guy into the financial domination fetish. He claimed "emptying himself out for me" would give him a tremendous erotic rush, then requested the name of my bank and account number to arrange this sexy wire transfer. But I cut off all contact with him, believing financial domination, commonly called "findom," was where women took advantage of men, not the other way around.

I initially only had a vague idea about findom, thinking it entailed either getting cash or receiving gifts from doting submissive men, in exchange for doing nothing but acting haughty and superior. I considered this an even better deal than being a pro-domme, where women received funds for *not* having sex with guys, just doling out some teasing and torture. (Cash or gifts given are always termed "tribute" by pro-dommes, findoms and the men who crave them.)

Unlike prostitution, with findom there's no sex involved. Like prostitution, there are funds involved. In stark contrast to the sticky icky intimacy hookers engage in, there is hardly any face time. In fact, most (but not all) findom is facilitated online.

As Clive had pointed out, I lacked both the strength and cruelty to be a proper slave owner, and would doubtlessly have the same limitations as a dominatrix. Could findom be a good fit for an adventuress in her sixties? As an incentive to post my own findom profile online, I completed an Amazon wish list, one mainly in the comfort shoe category. But these fellows were jonesing to buy young women six inch stiletto heeled sandals they could don to toy with or trample them. There was no way I could motivate any sub to buy a senior citizen the expensive Italian made orthopedic shoes she craved. Even so, I decided to investigate the world of financial domination.

Findom, like modeling, careers in advertising and becoming a pharmaceutical rep, was clearly the realm of the young'un. They called themselves brats or "princesses" and presented themselves as discerning, demanding and deserving. These fashion savvy girls knew the difference between what was chic and what was shit, and were ever ready to put a guy down for being a doofus while eagerly taking and spending his money. Submissive men, termed "pay pigs" or "money slaves" flocked to them. While a slave is erotically satisfied through serving and obeying commands, the *money* slave gets his rush through proving himself and providing.

There are pay pigs within the ranks of beta males and their alpha brethren. The beta believes he is a worthless loser, vastly inferior to all sorts of women. Those little rejections and romantic failures experienced as a geeky high schooler are ingrained in him—as an adult they're amplified. Money slaves aren't only found among working class males, loners or those with low self-esteem. There are wealthy or successful pay pigs who, though they hold themselves in high regard and have a positive sense of their worth, are erotically stimulated when hearing a woman say how useless and pathetic they are.

One such alpha male specified he was addicted to financial domination and spelled it out: "So-called princesses manipulate and prey on men who are made to feel inadequate." He described himself as a much lauded athlete those around him viewed as a role model. But there was something about this sexual transaction the athlete became addicted to. He would get online and spend a thousand dollars a night on just one findom, only to get nothing in return—except being told how his only purpose in life was giving her what she deserved. When in the moment, he found it erotically thrilling to hear how he's such a loser, especially coming from a woman who acted superior. But after he climaxed, he soon began to think for himself, then immediately regretted all that had transpired. Financial domination is now the only thing which gets his penis hard—as a consequence, he can't maintain his erection with regular girls. Findom is ruining him financially, not to mention destroying his life. He asserts it is a very insidious addiction, one difficult to stop.

Much of it is done by Russian gangsters and Nigerian scammers posting fake pictures of nubile young women in sassy poses, writing in their voices and assuming fictitious identities. There are scores of real life findoms all over the world and just as many fictitious ones. YouTube sensation Fetish Princess Amira appears highly suspect, and not only because she looks like a post-op transgender Middle Eastern mutt. Never speaking, she purses or licks her silicone inflated, fuchsia lips, blows cigarette smoke at the camera, bats the electric blue lids of her dark eyes and flashes the red painted soles of her high heeled shoes. (Showing someone the sole of your shoe is a huge insult in the Arab culture.) Though the Amira videos seem created by Middle Eastern men (crazed Arabian disco music accompanies many of her videos) her written message was in English, tailored to attract American male customers. Why else would this findom Scheherazade post so many videos with an American flag as the only backdrop? Even the name, *Amira*, which means princess in Arabic, points to Middle Eastern internet scam mayhem.

Just how would a guy find his way to Fetish Princess Amira's You-

Tube video? By internet searching the very thing that's distressing him—a financial domination addiction. Amira's headline reads: "Financial Domination Addiction...Sissies, Cucks, PayPigs, Let Me Help You!" In her written message, Amira initially appears understanding, expressing how a pay pig desires to be teased and controlled. The poor chump who has googled financial domination hoping for some help, now comes upon this Amira, who explicitly describes how it excites him to open his wallet and be used for his cash: "I know what it does do you, making you so weak, making your cock throb for more, you need to be used and you need to pay." Amira then enticingly promises spoiling her will become the guy's obsession. She next becomes demanding, claiming she deserves his money "so much more." The salient, realistic facts about the fellow's financial obligations (a wife and kids, debts, mortgages, loans, perhaps spousal or child support) are rarely addressed.

But Amira's YouTube viewers seem impressed: "On my kneeeeees," said one; "i'll eat ur smoke like a good pay piggy!" exclaimed another. "Thank you for letting me send You another tribute, Princess," an appreciative man wrote. Another fan agreed: "Easy to pay and worship but difficult to resist Her."

Though many men are in thrall to the media-driven concept of the perfect ten, most findoms appear as average looking women trading on a superiority complex. The only attitude a pay pig responds to is when the woman acts unobtainable, puts herself above him, and seems purely aspirational. These men are not interested in any woman who'd accept them in a romantic sense or would actually have sex with him. They'd rather masturbate to some domme's petulant phone chat while she insults or (even better) laughs at him.

Both findoms and pay pigs write internet posts much like personal ads, detailing exactly what they expect. Though the findoms have an elevated sense of self, those who seek them are realistic, both in how they view themselves and about what they are seeking. A guy will describe himself as a 54-year-old loser, or one who likes to be used and abused, both physically and financially. The pay pigs promise to be either money slaves or dedicated gift buyers for superior women and specify how they wish to be in a findom's life (mainly for her profit and pleasure). Their expectations are slim: they do not expect to have sex with their Goddess.

When a sub encounters a findom princess online, she usually throws out a line, one to reel in her pay pig. She'll not only promise to fulfill his every desire, but detail how she'll humiliate and degrade him. When she describes how she'll make him feel, it isn't the typical feel-like-a-real-man come-on. A findom is guaranteed to make her fellow regard himself as worthless and (even more exciting to him) rather stupid. Being called "dumb" won't offend this kind of guy; it is likely to give him the erection he craves.

Findoms are often in touch with one another, either bragging about their conquests or comparing pay pigs. One young findom described how she instructed a man to buy her an Apple computer. After he did so, she gloated to other findoms online about how she had "drained" him, then gleefully called him a retard and "pathetic old creep."

Most financial dommes call themselves findoms and don't beat around the bush about how they want to be viewed (as a goddess) or how they regard these males (as useless, worthless money slaves). Findoms insist they be worshipped and obeyed (not loved) and demand to be given everything they ask for. Even if they're not in their twenties, the typical findom will say she is; pay pigs find these young sugar babies irresistible.

A seasoned findom knows when a man craves being controlled. In such cases, she'll instruct her guy what to eat for each of his meals, including snacks and drinks. Not only will he be ordered how to dress and what to wear, every dollar he spends has to be approved by his findom first. A findom's end goal isn't merely being important to such a guy, it's running every single aspect of his life.

Their initial online come-on features the domme's picture; these range from partial nudity or kinky leatherwear to distorted head and shoulder shots. They display a countenance never friendly or serene but demanding, judgmental, or pouting—all contrived to convey a sense of bratty entitlement. In the mind of a sub, the princess he views online—

her thong stuffed with greenbacks and prominent posterior arched for his kiss—isn't just kinkster trailer park trash. This is his version of Gatsby's Daisy. These submissive men will, to a one, agree with her—she is a goddess.

Say a young woman had problems: she was laid off from her job, suffered a serious health crisis, got behind on the rent or her student loan. Even if she were the most fetching filly in all creation, money slaves never pony up for real need. Female desperation makes this kind of guy beat a hasty retreat. But if the same girl demanded money for frivolities (a sparkly new frock or the latest unnecessary electronic gadget) a pay pig will squeal with delight as he forks over the cash. The most successful financial dommes already have some form of steady income and treat what they make from subs as mad money.

Many women have turned to this uber-cynical findom career after a crushing disappointment in life. A dream was dashed, someone let them down, there was a failed romance with a vanilla fellow. Findom becomes their way to make sure it doesn't happen again—the guy must pay first and pay big to prove he is worthy of her time. "Calling All Losers!" bleats one findom's headline. A princess looking for a new cash cow will typically first complain, as if weary from and wary of any who'd waste her valuable time (meaning he'll not provide). Findoms are also known to scold potential suitors how they're not into game players or fakes.

Findoms often require their pay pigs to tribute before any further online contact, ensuring the domme won't remain empty-handed. Typical of these demands is the brat who instructs future suitors how a contribution to PayPal is necessary before serving her. This findom provides the necessary contact information, then waits for a fish to bite.

Willing guys typically respond as did this one: "You tell me, goddess, how much do I have to spend to earn your attention? It is an honor for me to work and give You all my money just to know You have a better life."

Findoms become familiar with the myriad varieties of pay pigs. One gets off sending several small payments to a variety of accounts, which are all controlled by that findom. Another becomes excited by how the amount owed is growing and growing. And then, there's everything in-between. Most tributes range from $50 to $750. Gifts received are often electronic items or designer purses worth many hundreds of dollars. But findoms realize a guy who tributes the greatest amount all at one time will be the one most likely to vanish. The working class hero, who goes without Starbucks so he can steadily send his findom $100 a month every month for several years, is deemed more valuable than a loaded fellow who sends $500 only once.

It's an arrangement where the submissive gets controlled by a woman he deems both desirable and deserving. (That's obviously not his wife!) For a dyed-in-the-wool pay pig, the prospect of having his chosen goddess dictate what he can and cannot spend, eat and purchase is a tantalizing one. The harsh reality—they're denying themselves and going without so they may spoil their mistress—brings a romantic, even erotic, dynamic into play.

The most effective financial dominatrices learn everything about their sub (what he owes, earns, all of his expenses) then tightens his spending. A hardcore pay pig reports every expenditure for his domme's approval. She'll have him on a budget; at the end of the month, half of what's left over can come her way. To the fellow who sexually responds to a cruel, greedy woman, this is exactly what he needs. He may have a wife and kids who love and depend on him—but providing for a bratty, demanding and controlling bitch is what drives him. The domme and her sub are constantly texting each other about his budget, cash intake and outflow. The fact he's never even met her is rarely seen as a red flag.

These transactions are facilitated through businesses which simplify gifting or transferring funds. A findom favorite is the Green Dot money pack. A pay pig will visit a store selling these money packs-for five bucks and provide the cashier with additional funds to load them. The eager fellow scratches off a strip which reveals a set of numbers. He e-mails these to his princess, who goes to another more privacy-oriented money site, enters the numbers her piggie sent and *voila*, the amount is instantly in princess' account, primed for her usage. Many findoms love Green Dot for keeping a guy at a distance, knowing her personal information is never disclosed. Other favored services include GiftRocket, Moneybookers (for guys outside the United States), the Payoneer debit card (which money can be loaded onto), and Web Pay.

When keeping tables on those seen as their property, a typical findom employs all the latest technology without compromising her anonymity. A findom will use Google voice to take/place calls or even text, never exposing her personal phone number. There are applications, primarily used for business, which can remotely access a money slave's computer to inspect all his personal files. One findom doyenne suggests pay pigs be controlled by changing his computer password and giving him a guest account, which limits the websites he can visit. She further recommends using his webcam to spy on him, copying any significant computer files, and obtaining his passwords to Facebook or even PayPal.

Because there are so many scam artists from all over the world presenting themselves as haughty female supremacists, and demanding big bucks for the privilege of being in contact with them, some pay pigs only respond to gift—not cash—requests. Most findoms are on Amazon or other shopping sites with registers and wish lists that could make a bridezilla envy their gall. Findoms who don't want to seem too cash greedy may list items such as expensive lingerie or luggage. The guys who give are quicker to gift; they imagine behind that beribboned box containing a Coach bag lies a real life dominant woman, one he will soon be in close contact with. (Certainly, this couldn't be a Ghanaian scammer masquerading as a domme, playing a cash cow for his hard earned wages!) And actually, these are (most of the time) independent young women actively finding men who'll buy them their every heart's desire. They often chat online with other findoms about their latest acquisition, courtesy of some hapless "Human Wallet." What is called *real time*, the pay pig's nirvana, hardly ever happens—his longed for abuse comes mainly from afar.

Then there is blackmail. If this fetish really pushes a submissive man's buttons, he'll usually allude to it; a quick witted findom will pick up the blackmail ball and run with it.

The domme gets her satisfaction knowing if he doesn't do what she says, he could be in jeopardy with his job, wife or kids. It's surprising to learn just how much personal information the pay pig will give a findom. Even relating something like when he last had sex with his wife can trigger a blackmail response, as in this example: "I have the date plus your wife's e-mail address and will act on this information if you don't perform exactly what I tell you to do." Findoms working the blackmail angle think they've painted their guy into a corner.

Most findoms display zero guilt and thoroughly enjoy what they do. In fact, they seem to be rather intoxicated when a man obeys them. Having a man perform exactly as she says is a findom's ultimate power trip. After the submissive male complies, many findoms experience a greater sense of self-worth and fulfillment, one which can last for days. Though the dommes' methods of connecting with the men and extracting tribute vary—as for their piggy prey, they all sexualize money and relish giving up control.

If I were about 40 years younger, would I be trying out the findom life? Or would I feel responsible for these guys and try to talk some sense into them? I wasn't ready to meet more slaves, and thought hanging out with a few harmless sissies or sissy maids would be a better fit. Yes, there is a difference between the two and neither are homosexual (though either can be bisexual). The *sissy* is a man who interacts with a dominant woman while feminized or being cross-dressed. The sissy *maid* desires to *serve* a dominant woman while he is dressed in female service attire. He sexualizes cleaning, housework and serving food or drink. Tea service (especially when done in a specific or ritualistic manner) is a major sissy maid fetish, as I learned at TES-Fest. Len, the first openly submissive man I encountered, had suggested he serve me tea while dressed as a female maid.

There are scores of closeted sissies and sissy maids who seek monogamy with an understanding female. Most of these guys think themselves good husband material. Just what do they have to offer—

besides sharing and adding to wifey's toiletries and wardrobe? As one sissy put it: "I am giving my special woman not only access to my secret world, but the authority that comes with keeping it strictly private." Not only do sissy wives have undeniable power over their husbands, such marriages typically have an unusually strong bond between the partners. Sissies and sissy maids view their wives as goddesses; they don't just put their partners first, but high upon the female superiority pedestal.

Anthony* was a suburban based sissy who was not into serving or doing chores—he was a *sissy* not sissy maid—but being submissive while dressed in women's clothes. This was, more or less, what he revealed on our first date. Anthony dressed well, had a lanky, fit frame and wasn't unattractive, just utterly nondescript. Seeing him again, this time dining out, I'd suggested a bag he'd checked be lugged back to my place. After returning from the restaurant, I poured him more wine. Anthony soon disappeared into my bathroom, where he changed into a pink camisole, black lacy bikini and patent leather high heeled pumps. Now feminized, he strutted and preened, admiring himself in my bedroom mirror, glancing down at his panty covered bottom and shapely calves. He donned no wig and wore no makeup.

He didn't want to be with a man and claimed never to have had any homosexual experience. Anthony's fantasies revolved around being dominated by a woman, all the while being dressed as one. How did he initiate being feminized and cross-dressed before he ducked into the bathroom to change? "Let's be girls together," he suggested in a seductive tone, while holding one of my hands. After coming out of my bathroom a changed man, I suggested perhaps we could paint each other's toenails. He chose a bright pink from among the several bottles I had on hand. The polish took just a few minutes to dry and Anthony was thrilled to be rendered even more girly.

He expressed his sexuality with trepidation. "Can I touch your breast?"

"Oh, sure," I replied, a bit too eagerly for him. As a submissive, it would have been more exciting to be denied with a sharp *no,* and maybe a slap. (This would have presented an opportunity to beg, which submissive men dearly love to do.) He hesitated before lightly, gingerly placing his open palm against one of my C-cups. I sensed his disinterest, as if this wasn't what he really wanted. There was no aggression, only trepidation. I remained seated while Anthony suddenly dropped to his knees and pressed his head between my breasts, as a small child would cuddle with his mother. That's what he wanted—not to act the sexual instigator, but to be the little boy again. There was no urgent sexual drive on his part, only a certain longing and distinct appreciation for womanliness.

"Is there any place you can sit where you're like...on a throne?" he asked haltingly.

"How about the Chinese Chippendale chair in the hall?"

"I noticed the chair—but can't stretch myself out underneath it, there's not enough space. I need to be lower than you."

After I had placed myself on my bedroom's electronic massage chair, he lay flat on the carpet near its foot rest, raising his torso in order to kiss, caress and massage my feet. "You have such lovely feet," he whispered. "Such slender toes." As he kneaded one foot, my other toyed with his bikini-clad penis. Wondering whether he was at all stiff, I could only feel the hardness of a device like an athlete's protective cup, certainly not any familiar jack-in-the-box male erection.

"I'm wearing the CB-6000," he offered in the prideful way of a new high-ticket sports car owner.

I was intrigued, as I'd heard so much about male chastity and the odd, sundry devices that caged the snake. At my request, Anthony pulled down his panties to reveal his polycarbonate and metal covered genitals. The thing made an odd appearance, provoking my curious cats to investigate and sniff about it. I couldn't stop gawking either, as I'd never seen anything quite like this. His flaccid penis was encased in a clear tube with each testicle forced to an opposite side. A sizable gold-tone padlock added an even more bizarre effect.

"Do you have a paper towel?" he asked. "You see, I'm leaking." Chastity devices put a kibosh on the male orgasm by stunting the wearer's erection. When such a man becomes excited, fluid usually dribbles out. The domme key holder refers to this event as a "ruined orgasm" and typically relishes in these frustrated passions. For subs who crave a woman to sexually control them, giving a special dominant the key to their locked up phallus is the answer. Those dominant women whose mantra is "control the orgasm, control the man" find satisfaction in being a key holder.

Anthony didn't need a key holder to don his CB-6000—he'd been wearing it non-stop for two weeks before we'd met. But it was his fervent desire to be with a dominant woman, one who'd understand how much he enjoyed orgasm control (plus the thing around his manhood). He maintained his chastity device was better than sex—wearing it provided a constant awareness which resulted in this low-grade, never ending stimulation.

He reported tremendous satisfaction in knowing he had a subversive secret which could easily be detected. "Just last week I was at work and had to use the urinals, where there were no dividers," he confided. "I became afraid someone coming in would notice my CB-6000, and was so nervous I was just shaking. Lucky for me, no one entered the men's room." He related another incident where a co-worker approached, suddenly hugged him, and immediately thereafter assumed a disquieted expression. Could she have noticed a certain bulky hardness? Anthony took pleasure in emerging unscathed from such close calls.

He liked to mention both his dick and his device, in the obsessive way I'd heard male porn stars talk about what they call their "moneymaker": *It's sore today; it needs rest; it needs Viagra; it's ready to work and can cut glass.*

"I need to stretch it out," Anthony related. There were other reports—"it's swelling," or "it's scraping." There was talk about how he needed to increase his penis's blood flow and more about how challenging the cage was to wear while urinating. As for the huge metal padlock he wore front and center, Anthony claimed he liked to keep it locked. The fact there was no female key holder present to control his orgasms didn't stop him—he liked wearing a self-locked chastity tool nonetheless.

I asked how long he intended to wear it. "Oh, I'm thinking like...forever," he replied in an impassioned voice. And typical of most men who were in chastity, he didn't have just one model, he had three.

As expected, a little begging was in order. "If I wear my CB-6000 for two weeks straight, will you let me have an orgasm? Please! Will you?"

"Sure!" I told him, though it was hardly what he wanted to hear. "When do you want to have an orgasm?"

"Maybe never," he muttered. He hung his head to avoid looking at me.

Such a posture deserves a collar, so I quickly retrieved one to place around his neck. After a leash was affixed to the D-ring, Anthony, who had been standing, instinctively dropped down on all fours. Eager to be led around that way, he approved the thick lace ribbon I tied around his entire plastic-encased, metal-adorned manhood. Now feminized, collared, leashed and in submission, he complacently crawled behind me. I needed to kick it up a notch by placing my homemade penis lead on his package. On his hands and knees, going from bedroom carpet to living room rug, now led by a rope attached to his locked away genitals, Anthony was in his bliss. I felt satisfaction in being able to read these subs, sense their particular needs (to be feminized, hurt, humiliated) then act accordingly.

Something told me he was ready to be taken to the next level—actually two things, both of his erect nipples—so I placed a small metal clamp on each. (Pin curl holders, bought from a beauty supply shop, served the purpose nicely.) His nips were plump and pointed between the little clips; I sadistically brushed my open hand about them for a more hurtful effect. Anthony was sufficiently excited to take a little pain and interpret it as pleasure, yet wasn't a hardcore masochist. He had me remove the clamps after about fifteen minutes, when he became aware they were making his nipples too sore.

This wasn't to be any slumber party, so I bid him goodnight and Godspeed back to the suburbs. He called me the next morning, asking when we could get together again, but I wasn't interested in seeing him further. He needed a key holder and inconveniently lived more than 90 minutes away from Manhattan. Although it wasn't practical on any level, the male chastity phenomenon had aroused my interest.

Scores of men have chosen to remain chaste—there are moral, religious, health or other deeply personal reasons to avoid having sex. For submissive men, wearing a chastity device is a desirable constant reminder of this restriction. I began viewing different models of male chastity devices, just to learn more about them. There have been chastity belts for women since the Renaissance. Penis cages for men were worn much later—one to prevent nocturnal erections and emissions was patented in 1909. The first male chastity device wasn't introduced until 1977. Actually called a "chastity apron," it was a clunky bulky thing compared to the breakthrough Protective Tube And Harness created in 2004 by Gines Sanchez Gomes. His invention, with its metal tube and padlock closure, was the prototype for all the others to come. Its purpose was baldly described by the inventor as "a method to assure masculine chastity."

Now created primarily from plastic or silicone, other models are composed of titanium and stainless steel. Though there are many different manufacturers of male chastity products, AL Enterprises dominates the field with its CB series. At any gathering of submissive men and the dommes they love, you'll hear them discuss the attributes and virtues of the CB-2000 or CB-3000 versus the CB-6000. Las Vegas-based AL Enterprises has been cranking them out for over a decade, with total units sold in the high hundreds of thousands. At a retail price point of between one and two hundred dollars for each schlong sheath, that's a lot of bucks to prevent the bang. Like the best-fitting pair of custom shoes, some high-end chastity devices are made to measure. There are models with trade names both fanciful (Queen's Keep, The Guardian, Watchful Mistress, Lancelot Classic) and descriptive (The Cage, The Tube, Buddy-Lock, and the Dickcage Duo).

I had previously assumed chastity devices were foisted on submissive males by their dominant female partners who'd had way too much of a good thing. Weren't women buying chastity belts for their guy as a way of saying "enough already"? (As I recalled, being involved with heterosexual men meant they were either always on you or plotting how to get in.) But I was wrong—buyers of chastity devices are overwhelmingly men who see it as BDSM lite. Having their dicks locked away is equivalent to perpetual bondage without the overt display of rope, leather and chains.

Dominant women who are involved with submissive men get a special thrill knowing their guy is frustrated, perhaps aroused, and can do nothing about it. Although dommes can crow about how their sub in chastity is "deprived" or made to "suffer for them," things aren't quite that way. For most submissive men, being in chastity is superior and preferable to penetrating a woman—with its end goal a seconds-long series of fuck fireworks. Chastity isn't about sensual deprivation for them, but can result in constant sexual awareness and stimulation, as Anthony had reported.

A fellow can urinate with the device attached; but when standing, if his penis does not fill the tube to the very end, or if the slot doesn't exactly line up, he's going to spray on the toilet. (Which could be a reason why his lady locked him up in the first place!) Whether to sit or stand, use a urinal or commode, it all makes for great debate among the chaste.

Now consider hygiene: a chastity device must be removed in order to wash the genitals. For this, you must have a key holder, a chosen female who is entrusted not only with the key but control over those genitals. The male chastity experience doesn't just revolve around their constricted appendage; it also involves that special lady given the power to release it. I've heard how "locking it away" produces intense feelings in subs towards their women, emotions more powerful than in men influenced by feminine beauty, youth or pure *amour*.

I'd be willing to see a man who wore a chastity device—but he'd have to live nearby, and our relationship would have to be intimate enough for the key holder dynamic to work. By the same standards I use with any vanilla fellow, Anthony wasn't right for me. I had mentioned to him, on more than one occasion, how my new printer needed setting up and why I wanted someone to do the installation with me. He was not at all interested in doing this, yet seemed tech savvy. I'd suggested painting each other's toenails; but after his tootsies were polished pink, he lost interest in the silver lacquer I'd chosen for my bare toes. There were a few more it's-all-about-me behaviors on his part. I was a broad-minded old broad, one who would date and entertain a sissy or man in chastity. But was this sub someone who would put me and my needs first, a man who truly catered to me? No.

SIXTEEN

The Pussycat And The Queen

I WAS NOW IN MY MID-SIXTIES, READY TO TRY ANY number of new things, ever mindful this was my last chance to so. Regretting how I'd long ago tossed away the hot pants I'd worn in 1971, I bought a similar pair of black wool shorts for the winter and, to go along, some over the knee boots. They weren't the iconic high heeled hooker boots worn by Julia Roberts in *Pretty Woman* but had low wedges—any footwear over two inches high now resulted in lumbar pain. Critically taking stock, I became increasingly aware a few more silvery hairs had cropped up in my pubic patch. If I didn't get an appointment for laser treatment now, I'd eventually be sporting Methuselah's gray beard between my thighs.

The technician at the laser spa had asked if I wanted to remove all hairs—and if not, how I wanted my pubes to appear. As a career pornographer, I'd seen the current styles, such as the narrow bit of vertical pubic hair called "the landing strip." I had even named a similar horizontal style "the Hitler mustache"—though my coinage never really caught on.

Replying to her question, I specified: "I think I want like a mullet. You know—business in the front, party in the back." She appeared nonplussed; I had to be more specific. "Just zap off all the hair around and below but leave the very top part, the mons Venus, alone. If it's totally bald, I'll just look like an ancient toddler and that's not where I have the gray hairs."

There was something irrevocable about laser hair removal, as with other trendy body modification methods. I'd noticed how many dommes had a few notable tattoos or piercings. But submissive men eschew body modifications and consciously strive to appear nondescript. They'll maybe shave their heads if balding or make their chests and backs hairless via razor, wax or laser (hair removal techniques used by many vanilla men, especially actors and athletes). While the dommes need to stand out, the subs seek to blend in.

The technician soon began to operate the laser device, which was much like first time sex—never accurately discussed when it hurts like hell. *If only I were a masochist like Spencer**. I always preferred people who were different, and he was definitely that. Spencer was an attractive accountant in his fifties. Although he identified as a submissive man, he presented as pure vanilla coated with an interesting layer of kinkster spice. Spencer didn't want to do chores, dress in women's clothing or be my slave. He was a stone masochist who welcomed CBT, ass walloping, and bondage along with various varieties of torment. He also responded well to a pinch of humiliation—but only when delivered with a dollop of pain.

Tall and muscular, Spencer made a favorable impression when we first met for lunch at an inventive Italian place I'd chosen. For our second date, we dined at one of my Pan Latin discoveries. Our third get together was his suggestion—a day at the beach, a local nude (or clothing optional) strip of sand. Sprawled on a beach blanket, I observed he was nicely hung and casually secure displaying himself in his natural state. Spencer had a serene self-acceptance which I found intriguing and undeniably sexy. Unlike a few other annoying subs I'd known, he didn't prattle on about high-powered women. As we lay together in the altogether, our naked skins warmed by the late afternoon sun, he revealed how he'd become a masochist.

Raised in a devout Roman Catholic family, he had attended a strict Catholic boys' school. There Spencer was made to watch church-sanctioned short movies on the lives of Saints. According to him, these filmed depictions of martyrdoms were so grisly and gory, the hyper-realistic, graphically detailed Mel Gibson crucifixion film, *The Passion of the Christ,* paled by comparison. Such scenes as the roasting of Saint Sebastian, Saint Bartholomew being skinned alive and Saint Hippolytus drawn and quartered were vividly etched in young Spencer's consciousness—along with the message such unimaginable suffering was not only joyful and satisfying for the martyred one, but God-approved. Or as Spencer remembered: "The tortured Saints were rewarded by God with things like stigmata, or more trials and adversity. Their agony was portrayed in such an exciting and positive way."

Spencer was also influenced by Saint Francis of Assisi—the way he had entered a fire without suffering burns, how he'd worn a hair shirt and frequently flagellated himself as penance. As a boy, he was also taught about all the Saints who practiced self-mortification. These were powerful role models for Spencer.

At both church and school, the specter of Christ's crucifixion was omnipresent. Priests and nuns repeatedly emphasized how Jesus had died for the sins of humankind, and greatly detailed the suffering and humiliation Christ had endured. Carrying his own cross, being spit upon by Roman soldiers, made to wear a crown of thorns, stripped of his robe, jeered at by a rowdy mob—it was all stressed daily. As a child, Spencer became fixated on the horrifying details of Jesus's crucifixion—how he was not only whipped but scourged, his side pierced by a lance, hands and feet nailed to a cross.

Young Spencer was not only a devout believer, he was a scared witless little boy. He'd been told (both at church and Catholic school) not to touch himself; and how doing so was a sin leading to eternal damnation. He'd heard what awaited sinners in Hell—and if touching down there led to an eternity down there, he wanted none of it. But at the age of six, Spencer was becoming all too aware of his penis, the very thing he had been warned not to touch. As a result, on several nocturnal occasions, he had tried to pull it off. One evening, this pulling resulted in what Spencer then thought was a very intense muscle spasm, but one he interpreted as an *ecstasy*—which he'd been taught was a rare, wonderful religious event.

Seeking more ecstasies, the precocious 11-year-old jerry-rigged a lawn mower motor so he could get off on its electric sparks. He also began tying himself—and his genitals—up in a variety of intricate ways. He'd affix a rope to his penis and throw the length over a ceiling beam to have a tug—an act young Spencer thought preferable to the sinful touching himself.

Spencer knew he wasn't like the other boys at school. By high school he'd read his behaviors were termed masochism and categorized as a mental illness, which greatly troubled him. He thought college fraternity membership would make him more normal—and became his chapter's sole pledge who secretly welcomed the paddle's whap. After an alcohol-soaked frat party, he bedded a co-ed who also liked to be stricken. Spencer kept his sexuality secret from all but her—they took turns whipping each other before having intercourse—and she became his girlfriend of many years. For Spencer, conventional sex was foreplay; true erotic satisfaction involved getting hurt.

His co-ed love continued her studies in another country and the couple parted. Spencer had spent the next few decades trying to find his perfect sadistic, dominant woman. I wondered whether it bothered him how I wasn't a natural, creative sadist or more of an instigator. But with his meaty rear wiggling before me, anticipating the first of many blows to come, it appeared as if that barely mattered. I had become comfortable with Spencer, having seen him a few times before even beginning to play. He'd brought a Bad Bag filled with his favorite toys and among them, various floggers. I chose a fringed model, one made from the inner lining of bicycle tires. Though it sounded impressively scary, I could tell by his unchanged skin tone it had made minimal impact. I tried another, this one made of nylon rope knotted at the ends. I then took in hand what Spencer called "a little smacker," a two-sided leather glove at the end of a stick. Next up was a single rawhide strip affixed to a plastic rod. Its narrow leather was "very stingy," he noted approvingly. With these new whamming and thwacking noises coming from the bedroom, one of my cats padded to the doorway and stuck her head in, just to investigate.

His reaction to the several consecutive whippings was enthusiastic. "Oh, wow, that smarts! Oh, yes, harder! Just hit it!" he begged, reminding me of how my college boyfriend would plead, "just suck it." Spencer's drive to be hurt was similar to a younger man's pent-up requirement for orgasm. After enough blows had been delivered and I stopped smacking his reddened buttocks, he straightened himself up, turned around, grabbed my hand and kissed it. "Thank you! That was just great!"

He'd slyly observed me in those moments between choosing the different flagellation devices and reported: "You had this glow. Your eyes were dilated and you were smiling. You loved it, and you're a natural!" A natural? Though I hardly agreed, I couldn't deny this warm and fuzzy feeling in a place where, only recently, I'd been rendered fuzzy no more.

Spencer, who was not really finished, then presented me with a thin wooden strip, one used to mix paint, and suggested I strike the head of his penis with this. As he held his phallus in both his hands and out to me, almost as an offering, he mentioned I should avoid the base of his genitals and be careful of the few bruises there. Hesitant as I was to do anything my homeowner's insurance didn't cover, I managed to deliver a few whacks to the head of his flaccid penis, and he finally seemed satisfied.

A savvy domme would never strike a hard on; penises can break or otherwise be damaged in the erect state. Neither would a savvy domme do any act her submissive requested—the dreaded "topping from the bottom" is a situation strictly to be avoided. But I was relatively inexperienced, usually welcoming feedback or suggestions. Spencer knew what he needed, and if it was something I was uncomfortable providing, it just wouldn't happen.

It mattered little to Spencer I wasn't terribly dominant—he wasn't deeply submissive. But those bruises troubled me enough to ask about them. "From some experiments at home," he casually replied. Receiving pain was how he expressed his sexuality. If he needed a release but there was no one around to hurt him, he'd do it himself. It was how he masturbated.

On another occasion, he'd had me inspect, then choose to use his breast press—its purpose was to put a submissive man's pectoral muscles in a vise. Two wooden parallel slats—one fixed, the other movable—came together via screws (which I initially had trouble threading). After his pecs were squashed in the press, I swatted them to heighten his excitement.

Spencer had an exceptional intelligence and a decent amount of self-respect. After we'd begun to see each other more often, I carelessly spoke about his masochism: "That's how you're wired."

"No, this is not how God created me," he replied with conviction. "I was made this way by the Catholic Church."

I liked to challenge him. "Children have a way of cutting through the baloney. They realize they have to go with the program; but sooner or later, if something is bullshit, they figure it out. Sounds like you were a bright little boy. Why'd you buy into it?"

"It was mainly because of Santa Claus." It wasn't that Spencer objected to the commercialization of Christmas—but how, as a youngster he was told Santa was all-knowing, and if you were good he'd reward you with presents. For a six-year-old, seeing is believing. "After several good Decembers, why would I doubt anything else—like going to Hell for touching myself? Or that physical suffering is not only virtuous and noble—but would guarantee me a place among the angels. So, how did you learn there was no Santa Claus. How old were you?"

"When I was in kindergarten, my mother informed me Santa was a complete fabrication—but warned me not to share this information with my little Christian friends or I'd get a spanking."

"Did you hear the other kids go on about what Santa might bring them at Christmas?"

"Sure, I listened for many years. I didn't give anything away to my schoolmates and tried to act enthusiastic, asking what Santa brought them, even when I knew Christmas morning was being staged by their parents." I also remember feeling distant, removed and always observing, while keeping my thoughts to myself. People never really change all that much.

I asked Spencer if he thought the experience was his alone, or whether the Catholic Church of 50 years ago was a veritable petri dish for subs. "You definitely get conditioned by them," he declared. "Look at the practice of confession, designed to elicit a feeling of excitement and humiliation. You're telling all your sins and secrets to someone in a position of authority you can't see—and the priest has no response but for a set and predictable absolution." Although Spencer believes he's one of many masochists created by a strict Catholic boyhood, I knew of just as many Protestant and Jewish men eager for any pain or humiliation a dominant woman can dish out. (I encountered several Jewish subs due to the one million plus Jews in New York City.)

It is a fallacy to think masochists interpret pain as pleasure—their pain is felt as just that. But a masochist processes pain in a different way, so he may get high. It's well known how adrenaline is immediately produced, to quickly course through the body when one is surprised, angry or threatened. But say you've not just been fired, and your adrenaline comes from a domme's cane striking your backside. As soon as you realize you *want* this caning and there's no cause for alarm, your brain can easily continue making adrenaline. This kick is just the start, but important to have, as you need that adrenaline rush to produce endorphins.

Everyone has heard how endorphins, the hormones responsible for our moods, are created when running, or produced (in smaller measure) by eating chocolate. Endorphins can work as natural painkillers as well and arrive several minutes after the first production of adrenaline. (Spencer had mentioned "getting warmed up for more extreme action," which is why I'd first whip or flog him a while.) Once endorphins are on the scene, now comes this physiological fork in the road. A subconscious decision is made either to orgasm or go for a euphoric high. (More specifically, the choice is whether or not to make a certain hormone which unleashes the sex hormones—or continue producing endorphins to reach a trance-like state.) Those masochists who choose not to come but go with the flow, report their reflexes slow and everyday logic somehow disappears. This spaciness lasts far longer than an orgasm (typically about a dozen seconds) and can result in a delicious bliss or feeling of ecstasy, one which may go on for hours. That is Spencer's happy place and he likes being hurt, if it's the way to get there.

He also made me consider the word *passion,* and its fascinating etymology. For most of my life, I had thought this word signified eroticism or strong emotion—totally unaware of the fact *The Passion,* when capitalized, referred to the crucifixion of Jesus Christ. (I first learned the word *passion* is from the Latin *passio*—which means to suffer—reading reviews of Mel Gibson's 2004 biblical epic *The Passion of the Christ.*)

While I was seeing Spencer, I was also being served by a sixtyish Manhattan slave, Phillip*. Phillip was a partner in his own business alongside his ex-wife, with whom he had two grown children. Throughout their long marriage and on several occasions, he'd tried getting his wife to lead. He specifically told her how he wanted to serve her, follow her instructions, have her make all the decisions—but she would have none of it. Though he took her to a meeting of a local BDSM organization, The Eulenspiegel Society, it failed to ignite any interest on her part. Phillip's wife wanted the man to take charge, as most traditional women do. And she strictly forbade her spouse from seeing any dominant women.

Believing his wife was inhibiting his life, Phillip filed for divorce and began seeking out service situations. The competition, those many other male subs vying to serve, was daunting—but he eventually became a car sub to a mistress in her late fifties. Every Wednesday he'd pick up this domme outside her Manhattan apartment and drive her for a day of suburban shopping. He'd wait for her at the Costco, outlet mall or wherever she wanted to go, before she reappeared, demanding he drive her home. Over several years of service, he wasn't encouraged to visit her residence and there was little interaction between them. As for any physical dominance and submission, it never happened. For three years, until the domme moved out of the area, Phillip continued to drive due to his drive—his strong need to serve a woman.

He also found a domme in her early sixties who ordered him to clean her home. There he swept, scrubbed, and dusted—again, with no real relationship. One day, this arms-length arrangement shifted. As Phillip vacuumed her rug, the mistress silently approached from behind, reached over and gave his nipple an unexpected, cruel little tweak. He was surprised and became aroused, though it was the beginning and the end of anything personal between them. According to Phillip, this sudden aggressive action and the submissive feelings it stirred in him revealed all that was possible. He maintained his divorce, the disruption of his family, and the damage to his business-partner wife was all worth it—just so he could experience being a servant.

I was surprised to hear he'd initiated divorce proceedings, as he seemed so extraordinarily passive. Any sexual urges he may have had were either suppressed or nonexistent. But this was not uncommon. Another submissive man had told me how, as a young man, he was finally alone with a woman he desired, someone he was wildly attracted to. After disrobing, she'd instructed him to "ravish her"; but he could not even begin to do so. He had to be told—actually, *ordered*—exactly what to do.

On a few occasions, slave Phillip had come by, helping me to do chores or the laundry. Immediately after entering my door, he'd drop to his knees and prostrate himself before kissing my feet. The man wasn't merely personable, but possessed a particular vibrancy. Although he liked to bow his head and avoid direct eye contact in my presence, this slave was not one to fade into the background. When I asked about his experience and learned about the mistresses he'd served, I couldn't comprehend his investment in women who'd used him so cavalierly.

One day, after he'd worked doing my laundry and cleaning windows for four or five hours straight, I prepared a very casual meal. (He'd confided those other mistresses had never fed him during or after his hours-long duties.) Slave Phillip seemed uncomfortable as I dished out soup and slung some readymade salad on a plate. "Shouldn't I be serving you, madam?" Of course. But it was my kitchen, I knew where everything was, and thought it easier to do it myself. After we sat down to eat, it bothered him that we were on the same level; he would consume no food unless he dined on the floor. My natural friendliness often made him recoil. Although I saw him as a person, that creature-livestock thing is precisely how he wished to be regarded. For this reason, Phillip quickly lost interest in serving me.

Though slave Clive had advised me to "treat them mean to keep them keen," it hadn't sunk in. For most submissive men, it is not a woman's beauty or personality which keeps them coming back for more—it's their selfish, bitchy behavior or sadistic skillset. The most active and popular lifestyle dommes are neither young, pretty, slender nor particularly successful, but are the strictest.

As a teenaged girl, my mother never taught me how to cook, clean or iron (she did no housework) and didn't expect me to perform any domestic duties. Instead, she told me "how to handle the maid." As a consequence, I was a fairly household helpless adult. But as a sixty-something domme, I now found myself dredging up Mother's advice and applying it to my slaves. What did Mommy say? "Make sure they know who's boss. Never seem insecure or unsure of yourself—it makes them uncomfortable. Never let your guard down and allow them to see you as a person with problems. And don't get too friendly with them."

I realized all of this gradually, and by the age of 65 had several submissive men serving me. These chore boys weren't choir boys but would eagerly clean the refrigerator, rearrange my household supplies, run errands and generally do my bidding so long as I was distant, demanding, and aloof. Their only reward was some occasional physical cruelty and I never fed them (as I did my cleaning lady). I was constantly on guard—if I appeared to be kind or understanding, it would only be perceived as weakness and my sub would soon disappear.

I'd had my sissy experience with Anthony, but thought being served by a sissy maid, and not just a sissy, was worth investigating. The sissy maid may cross-dress, but he's either bisexual or (more often) heterosexual. I saw several sissy maids at TES-Fest and had spoken to one right after my return from NELicon. Where an Adult Baby seeks to be taken care of, the sissy maid only wants to take care of his lady. That's why I wanted to check out Luke*, a preppy executive by day and preening sissy maid by night. A divorced man in his forties, Luke began our phone conversation by describing his Manhattan apartment, as would someone looking for a roommate. "It's a unique live-in opportunity where you'd have your own bedroom—the master of course—with a private bathroom. I'm in a luxury building. But within those walls, I would actually be your enslaved maid, serving only to pamper you. I do all the traditional wifely duties like cooking, cleaning, laundry and ironing. My lady would only require one thing of me—deep feminization requiring me to think, look, dress and behave like a wife or maid. I accept my purpose in life is to serve the deserving female, make her life more pleasurable. So, are you a girl who would be comfortable training me for strict obedience, a girl who enjoys feminizing men?"

"No, I'm not a girl. I'm a woman a lot older than you." It soon became clear my advanced years had rendered me undeserving of his kinky attentions. I immediately thought of my friend Candy, a vanilla woman yet natural dominant, who was ten years younger than I. She was then out of work and ever eager for a wealthy boyfriend. I imagined she'd be up for living large, all the while being served and spoiled by a man dressed as her slutty sister. "Although we're not a good fit, I can talk to my much younger friend and perhaps arrange an introduction."

Luke wanted to know the age of my friend, emphasizing how anyone a day over forty was unacceptable, even if she looked much younger. He groused about how he had always gotten introduced to different young women; but now, no one he knew would fix him up. I asked him why, and, since perhaps he now regarded me as a motherly type, Luke unloaded his tale of woe, or how his feminine service fetish had endangered his livelihood.

Just a few years ago, it had seemed as if all Luke's same-aged friends were getting married. To keep up with his peer groups—at work, or from college and his private club—he felt he should wed as well. He had often agreed to meet his co-worker's sister or a client's best friend from school. And why not? The Ivy League educated Luke was close to the Manhattan male ideal.

Not only did he eventually marry a woman from within his social circle, Luke's new bride also worked in his field. She was from a wealthy family who'd paid for a grand wedding, one attended by hundreds of well-wishing friends and colleagues. He'd settled on this particular miss as she seemed both sophisticated and understanding—the woman most likely to accept his sissy maid fetish and keep it their own little secret. What wife wouldn't like being pampered and waited on, he rationalized. During the first few months of their marriage, she didn't pick up on the few little hints he left. But one day he just sprung it on her. When Luke's bride saw him wearing his wig, maid's uniform, XXL fishnet hose, and size fifteen high heeled black leather pumps while fricasseeing the chicken, she bolted, never to return.

She instead consulted a divorce attorney. Although they'd had a pre-nup, because of what she knew about him, this wife clearly had the upper hand, both in the separation agreement process and in the dissolution of the marriage. But what really crushed Luke was the way she had clued in all of their pals why she'd left such a promising union, and exactly how they were not the perfect couple.

"I saw some friends of hers in a restaurant just last week. When they also noticed me there, I saw them put their heads together to whisper, then break up in laughter. I knew it was about me, not that I can do a damn thing about it. And, of course, they talk to my business associates. So whenever I enter a room, do any deal, I'm always wondering what they know, what have they heard? These thoughts fill me with such anxiety, it's affected my ability to function in the workplace. So, the lesson learned is clearly not to get involved with anyone I already know. I thought a mistress would be more understanding—but not someone a lot older than I am!"

Now realizing I should be seeing men nearer my age, I contacted a Manhattan-based sissy maid just a little over sixty. When we spoke, he had emphasized how I should not allow him to have what he called "the erections most of my gender thrive on." He also declared he would not show any erotic interest in me. Instead, his sex drive would be reconfigured by the immaculate cleaning of my home, while wearing a black maid's frock with matching white lace trimmed bonnet. But we were never to meet. I had two cats, he claimed to be extremely allergic, and it was not the way he wanted to be punished.

Men who sexualize house cleaning took notice (at an early age) of someone, probably their mother, doing household chores. A male's fetishes become imprinted on his subconscious mind at around six years old, or during their first stirrings of sexuality, and are triggered by something they've seen. One sub I met had noticed little girls wearing scarves when he was around that age. As a consequence, he eroticized scarves for the rest of his life. The man was hopelessly drawn to both sturdy head-wrapped babushka broads and those svelte, chic chicks with silk scarves draped and tied about their swan-like necks. When he's in bondage, he craves a woman to secure him by tying a silk scarf around his wrists or ankles, then slither one about his nipples before wrapping another around his member.

The classic example of a lifelong fetish first sexualized when a child is the foot fetish, often accompanied by a love of legs, shapely calves and high heels. My friend Jana Krenova, the preeminent leg fetish photographer, explained how the pre-school aged boy often sprawls at his standing mother's feet and looks up, feeling dominated, perhaps helpless, and sometimes fearful of being punished or abandoned. More commonly, he could simply feel a sense of adoration for his mother. But these are all strong emotions that can be internalized, left to develop and much later, years after puberty, manifest in a major fetish. Notwithstanding the males who appreciate how a woman walks, stands or looks in a tight skirt when wearing high heels—there are also guys who want to feel those high heels digging into their scrotum. He will lie in the supine position before a domme just to feel her stocking-clad calves tighten about his awestruck face, squeezing his slack-jawed mouth shut in submission.

A number of men have very specific, odd fetishes. One sixtyish man wanted a mistress who drove her sub wild by wearing her hair in an up-do. When I spoke with him, he detailed his preference for women who wore bouffant versions of French twists and beehives. "Your hair should be intricately done and heavily sprayed, because hair lacquer really drives me crazy." When I asked him if it was his mother who wore the beehive, he became indignant. How dare I accuse him of having incestuous thoughts! No, he confessed a little later, the big hair belonged to his aunt.

Guys with fetishes were my stock-in-trade—yet I refused to see any sub or slave who was wed or otherwise attached and nixed anyone who described himself as gay or bisexual. (It's difficult enough dating as a 65-year-old; doubly so when your prospect prefers a same sex sweetheart.)

Even after applying such strict criteria, I had scores of attractive fellows available to follow my orders, take me out or accomplish tasks. On one occasion, I'd told my friend Suze I couldn't make plans for a certain day—I had a slave coming over to help me retrieve several coats from the furrier (where they'd been in cold storage over the summer). Afterwards, the slave and I would rearrange my shoe closet—he'd also use duct tape to repair some boot boxes' ripped corners. When she asked what kind of action the fellow was receiving in return, I explained there was absolutely no sex (and certainly not affection) involved. I didn't have to get into any weird scene—the guy just wanted to *serve*. Suze was stunned and though not entirely disbelieving, could not comprehend such an arrangement. When she asked me if I had a favorite, I confessed how they were much like my preferred Manhattan restaurants—some were worth a return visit, but it was mainly all about the new or next one.

She had also wrongly assumed submissive men could not achieve an erection, which is hardly the case. The very act of their submission often gives them a serious stiffy. Whether they are allowed to orgasm (or not) is entirely up to their domme. And if their unit can hold up during penetration is a question I can't answer. The vast majority of submissive men do not crave penetrative sex and I've never had intercourse with a submissive man.

I confided in Suze how servants could come and go; but the only man I wanted to see again was one who did no chores, the masochistic Spencer. Naturally, she asked if I thought we had any "future." Seeing his initial embroidered after mine on our bath towels was never anticipated, although we got along well enough and he usually deferred to me. Even if he would consider my word as law and always endeavor to please me...who was I kidding? I wasn't really looking for someone; I was always looking to see what someone would do next.

And in that way, Spencer managed to hold my interest. But were we compatible? Not really. Although he was impressively hung, I was not impressed that he used his appendage for penetrative sex. The man was nearly vanilla! I told Spencer I'd consider it some time in the future—but only if I tied him up first so he could be ridden. There would be no mounting of me; but if he were in bondage, I'd control any thrusting. Subs don't usually go in for intercourse—they perform "body worship" or "queening."

I'd just recently bought a queening stool on eBay; but it was not to be used with those men I call Tongue Waggers, who I avoided like a virus. (And yes, a woman can get HPV or Human Papilloma Virus from a tongue, which typically contains more germs than a penis.) The typical Tongue Wagger is an older fellow whose flag now flies at half mast. He compensates by developing a tongue able to flick faster than the beating of a hummingbird's wings. Guys who suffer from premature ejaculation syndrome usually have their Tongue Wagger degree, *cum laude*.

A typical Tongue Wagger would probably be Jason*, a man who referred to himself as a "cum slave." Jason offered hours of what he termed "oral service" and promised so many multiple orgasms I'd have trouble seeing straight. There are many like him who may say they're slaves and identify as submissive but are actually nothing of the sort. Their sense of self-worth is derived from a particular orgasmic prowess, always delivered through digits, tongue, and toys—never the phallus.

These subs immediately lead with sex—posing questions about erotic performance and preferences. They can get a foot in the door by offering to clean, and typically prefer to do their chores in the altogether. But shortly after their nudie duty, it's on to the pooty. Hardly authentic submissive men, these oral-driven guys seek to control women through a highly developed ability to give orgasms. Even with zero oral prowess, if he raises the subject of vibrators or brings along a big toy bag of buzzers, similar motivations are suspect.

I remembered the experience I had under my canopy bed with Mister Slave. He certainly had that technique, but it was matched with an appealing, non-threatening, as-you-wish servile attitude. The Tongue Wagger is eager to please only sexually—not even close to servile in demeanor—and can be demanding. These are not authentic submissive men but sex addicts seeking to control women through cunnilingus. When a dominant woman begins to buck her torso, flail her limbs or involuntarily trill in orgasm, his ego is validated. He has deemed her, for the moment, either out of control or controlled by *him*. In the mind of a Tongue Wagger, he has rendered a powerful woman helpless.

Far from being a Tongue Wagger, the masochistic Spencer was never that annoying, sex-forward guy and proved to be a sensuous lover. When taking one of his thick nipples between my lips, hearing him urge me to bite them was a novel experience. I did so—gently at first, then much harder. I imagined I was getting too rough, thought he might be sore the next day and told him as much. "Don't worry about it," he muttered, between appreciative moans. "Just don't bite them off."

It almost goes without saying how when a person wants a partner to hurt him, there should be a certain level of trust. The same can be said for pleasure. One night, I changed into some vintage lingerie and lay face down on my bed so Spencer could massage me. He knew how to administer expert back and foot rubs, liked to give me pleasure and hear my satisfied groans. I thought Spencer the perfect sub with whom to break in my queening stool. At age 65, if I didn't have new experiences *now*, then when would I?

His eyes widened as I brought the strange looking leather bench out of my bedroom closet and patted the rug beside it. "Here's where you lie down." I used that firm but feminine tone subs respond to and put the padded head rest beneath my new purchase. Submissive men are drawn to women who please themselves first. Without the least bit of trepidation, Spencer lowered himself on the floor and lay his head on the leather pad, inside the stool's open area. I lifted the skirt of my vintage John Kloss nightie and plopped down on the thing, noticing how it automatically opened one's vagina for action—yet his tongue couldn't reach me. I'd sat down as I would on a chair, having had no idea a queening stool must be mounted cowgirl style, rear forward. But he had almost immediately figured that out—after which I turned around and the cunnilingus or queening commenced.

The difference between queening, facesitting and smothering is a subject for debate among BDSM devotees. (These words describing cunnilingus are similar only as they involve a woman who assumes the superior position.) Queening or facesitting happens when a dominant woman sits on or straddles a male's upturned face and rubs her genitals against the mouth and/or nose of her sub. Smothering involves cutting off your submissive partner's intake of air by placing—not poising—those naughty bits over his nose and using full weight body pressure. I loved-how the word *queening* also refers to giving birth...for kitty cats.

The act of queening was known in several ancient cultures, including Indian and Chinese. It was even depicted in Egyptian hieroglyphics. Queening was typically practiced by upper class women who sat on their orally skilled slaves' faces in order to achieve orgasm. In old Japan, there were brothels where male slave prostitutes served women this way.

Queening did not originally convey an evil measure of girl power. It was done by young maidens who had to retain their virginity, and perhaps demonstrate it with a wedding night bloody sheet. It took place among randy wives, whose husbands were off at war or on crusade, women who could not risk getting pregnant. Though queening was practiced by women from many cultures and during several periods of history, it only satisfied upper class ladies—those who regularly bathed, had time for pleasures and ruled their roost. Though cunnilingus is now a widely practiced sexual act, few women own queening stools; they are only used by BDSM devotees.

Submissive men like to "worship at the altar," an expression they often use to mean performing oral sex on a woman. A queening stool puts submissive men in their place, well below a woman, while he services her and brings pleasure. Dominant women find this low seat a magical open sesame for sex—it makes the pelvic floor muscles relax and the labia minor more exposed for maximum arousal. Submissive guys love it because it is both impersonal and humiliating. There are no sweaty body parts coming together and no female flesh to be caressed or randomly grabbed. It renders a man the more passive participant, and limits the level of intimacy while engaging in this most intimate act.

My queening stool experience was more about female empowerment than sexual ecstasy. It complemented my habitual detachment, while still being great fun. And I liked feeling on top and in control. Was I the sadistic female supremacy bitch goddess slave Clive craved? Hardly. But there are several ways a woman may express her dominance, from FLR's (Female Led Relationships) to the most severe consensual slavery. As Master Peter had remarked at the slavery workshop I attended, the line is where you draw it.

I gazed at the sight behind me—a man stretched out on my bedroom rug, his head disappeared beneath my seat. *If this is where they think they belong, that's where I'll put them.* One of my curious cats perched on the bed nearby, contemplating us with an unflinching, clear-eyed gaze as I sat on my quirky little leather throne.

A HEADPRESS BOOK
First published by Headpress in 2015

{t} 0845 330 1844 {e} headoffice@headpress.com

MISTRESS PUSSYCAT
Adventures With Submissive Men In The World Of Femdom
an invesigative memoir

Book design & layout: Ganymede Foley
Cover layout: Mark Critchell
Headpress diaspora: David Kerekes, Thomas Campbell,
Caleb Selah, Giuseppe, Dave T.

A CIP catalogue record for this book is available from the British Library

ISBN 978-1-909394-25-4 (paperback)
ISBN 978-1-909394-26-1 (ebook)
NO ISBN (hardback)

Headpress. The gospel according to unpopular culture.

The NO ISBN special edition hardback of this book, and other items, are available exclusively from World Headpress

1 HEAD PRESS EST 1991

WWW.WORLDHEADPRESS.COM

Lightning Source UK Ltd.
Milton Keynes UK
UKOW06f1015020915

257901UK00001B/24/P